Die Dieting?

OR

Lose Weight Permanently

Don Paullin

LifestyleWeightExperts.com

Lifestyle Weight Experts

Permanent Weight Loss™

Die Dieting? or Lose Weight Permanently. Copyright © 2010
By Don Paullin. Published by Business Certification
Publishing, Inc.

ISBN: 978-0-9785314-5-4

Printed in the United States of America
Publication Date: August 2010

Cover and interior property of Lifestyle Weight Experts, Inc.
Cover design by Bill Burnett
Interior book design and layout by: Lightning Source
Inc./Ingram Content Group

Business Certification Publishing, Inc.
Box 610

DIE DIETING OR
LOSE WEIGHT PERMANENTLY

You Will Learn Why:
- Lifestyle is the Only Path to Permanent Weight Loss
- Baby-Stepping Lifestyle Changes Work Permanently
- Best Keys for Your Lifestyle Changes to Best Bod
- Dieting Fattens You Instead of Flattens You
- You Gain Dieting Weight After Losing Dieting Weight
- Focusing on Weight Loss Assures Weight Gain
- Dieting Causes Wallet Loss & Rebound Pounds
- Before and After Pictures Sell You Again & Again
    1. Body, Mind, and Spirit Musts for Permanent Weight Loss
    2. Lifestyle Thoughts Can Make You Fat Ugly or Hot Bod
    3. Changing Lifestyle Self-Talk Changes Jeans Size
- Increasing BB Decisions Kicks Dieting's Ass
- Can Cans that Don't Expire Before You Do
- Processed Foods Cause Fat Ugly Depressions
- Lifestyle Eating Naked is Fun and Life Thinning
- Scales and Calorie Count for Weight Gain

It All Starts with the Body, Mind, and Spirit
Fat Warriors believe that your mind is the most powerful tool you have to regain your Right Size. Sometimes you must lose your current mind to find your positive mind. You could argue that you

need the Body, and you could argue the Spirit is key. Fat Warriors believe the trilogy of Body, Mind and Spirit (BMS) may be all one. We're not sure about that, but we are sure of one thing: BMS is left out of most diet plans and that is why they fail.

Look Great, Feel Great, Get a Date
We will show you powerful ways to use your mind to win your Beautiful Bod (BB). In fact, it will tie your Body, Mind, and Spirit together to access powers you may not know you had. That is the goal of Fat Warriors – to empower your trio of BMS so that you own and control your lifestyle for happiness, looks and health. You will also understand why diet plans fail you and cause rebound pounds. You will not use before and after pictures for proof, but rather your own judgment. *"Does this make common sense to me? Then I will do it."* You are the judge and jury of what is right for you and nobody else. You are in total control of your lifestyle. You can demand your Best Bod and get it. It is not about weight loss or gain, it is about a better life and happiness. It is for YOU and about YOU.

Fat Warriors focus is on gaining, not losing.
Gain what you desire!

ACKNOWLEDGEMENTS

I must thank all the profitable diet plans whose failures demanded I write this book. I was especially inspired by their quick and easy guarantees, plus the bonus of before and after pictures. These gimmicks do not work for permanent weight loss, which was my motivator to write this book. My special thanks to:

Trish Boos, who not only fought through the maze of my writing, but inspired me to dig deeper. She worked her editorial magic to help make my wandering writings into organized pages called a book. Thanks for being my all-purpose contributor.

Kay Reissig. Kay has become my personal friend, loyal confidante, and drill sergeant. Kay sets a work ethic example, and gives us the boot to work a little harder and deliver a little quicker (she is little).

Mary Jane Scott, who boots our Boot Camps up, edits and does whatever it takes. I am also glad she is my special friend.

Casey Karl, for his social media insights.

Kandi Amelon, for her fresh ideas and feedback. Her ideas were used in both of my books.

Dick Juntunen. Dick has been a good friend who has helped me in all my works.

Vicki Paullin, who made me believe I could be a writer.
Jason Shaw. Jason creates videos and sets them to music to take on video life.

Also, special thanks to: **Marianne Phelan, Isabel Clop**, and **Ted Dawson**.

This book was written with coffee bean stimulation provided by the wonderful baristas at Starbucks and Caribou Coffee. Thanks people. And beans!

DISCLAIMER

This book is based on the behavioral expertise of Don Paullin of Lifestyle Weight Experts' Fat Warriors program. It is based on behavioral and lifestyle change principles. We will not sell you pills or expensive plans. You can follow the Fat Warriors program for minimal cost and it will pay off in huge, non-fattening dividends of smiley pride.

This book does not take the place of medical help provided by physicians and other professionals. **Our Lifestyle Weight Experts' advice is based on the principles of behavior and lifestyle changes that will win for you.**

Our presumption is that to follow this book you must have the basic judgment and education to know what is best for you. We are presenting a new and unique approach. Lifestyle Weight Experts' program requires a paradigm shift of thinking that differs from easy, quick programs and miracle diets. Programs with before and after pictures seem to be right for those pictured, but never seem to work for anyone in achieving permanent change. If the pictures are your motivators, then stop reading and go take pictures. The Lifestyle Weight Experts Program may not be right for everyone, but it may be right for *you*. You decide.

Nothing in this book is based on diets, plans, or pills. It seems that most diets, diet plans, and pills fail, and are nothing other than clever marketing gimmicks. The Lifestyle Weight Experts Principles are based on common sense, and this book is completely different from others you will find on the topic.

So read, laugh, smile, cry, think, and then put on your War Face, growl, and fight fat!

TABLE OF CONTENTS

CHAPTER 1

YOUR PERMANENT LIFESTYLE FOREVER HOT BOD?

Lose Your Fat Can

You have come to the Lifestyle Weight Experts' Fat Warriors program driven by hope that we just might be something different that works. You are motivated by pain and desire to change from sad Fat Ugly to happy Hot Bod. You are skeptical and disbelieving because diets and programs have failed you. You are skeptical and don't believe anything will work. Being wrong is sometimes good news. You *can* lose your fat can for good!

Fat Ugly

Fat is not just fat, it is ugly. Fat metastasizes. It attaches to your face, butt, stomach, thighs, and sticks to you everywhere until it overwhelms your Beautiful Bod (BB) and becomes Fat Ugly (FU). If you are fat, think of your image to yourself. Think of your image to others, to the dating community, the matrimonial scene. Do people compliment you? Do they say your dress (or tent) is beautiful, that you have such a pretty face, or that's a great belt around your great waist? Now your Fat is an Ugly sight, where do you go?

It is important that you understand that *you* are not personally Fat Ugly, because the beautiful person inside you is surrounded on the outside by layers of imprisoning fat. **Your BB is inside the FU layers and crying for help to get out.** The beautiful person who resides inside is sending pounding brain signals of

1

painful depression, avoidance, health issues, and feeling horrible 24-7, hoping to be heard and freed. The beautiful person inside wants out!

You See It Everywhere

Your BB or FU Bod is on display everywhere. You drive your Hot Bod or Fat Ugly Bod around and it is seen at the store, at work, at play, and on the beach. Fat Warriors believe that there are no fat people, but rather beautiful bodies we have been graced with and should love. The problem is that these Beautiful Bods sometimes become immersed and surrounded by fat. It is these imprisoning layers of fat that hide your BB that we call Fat Ugly or FU. Do not think of FU as anything else but Fat Ugly that is hiding your Beautiful Bod and making you sad all the time. We will help you kick Fat Ugly's ass right off you so you can show off your new healthy Hot Bod.

Defining Fat Ugly

If it looks like a duck, then it's probably a duck. Look at your waist, butt, and under-arm flab, and you will know Fat Ugly when you see it.

Your Right-Sized Bod is inside of you. You have just covered it, layered it, and smothered it with Fat Ugly. You have hidden it until your Beautiful Bod can't be seen. You just need to remove the Fat Ugly camouflage to see it. We want your FU lost and your BB back.

The great news is that you can free your Beautiful Bod, but you must pay the price and make lifestyle changes to become your Hot Bod best.

Fat Ugly Life Sentence for Me?

Reality is that being Fat Ugly for most is unhealthy, embarrassing, unsexy, and a self-esteem killer. How long your BB is imprisoned by Fat Ugly depends on YOU. If you do not change your lifestyle, are you willing to serve a Fat Ugly life sentence?

2

Fat Warriors believe that you are a BB! Not to be shot from a gun, but rather a Beautiful Bod that you can love and show the world. Your BB belongs to you and you deserve it. So decide to take it back and you will do it. Yes, you can!

You are probably confused at the name calling. Is it Hot Bod, Best Bod, Beautiful Bod, or does it matter?

Fat Warriors Have Declared War on Fat in America!

Fat Warriors do not promote skinny, but we are at war to defeat Fat Ugly and win your Beautiful Bod. The goal is a new lifestyle that results in attaining your personal Right Size and a happier, healthier you.

Fat Warriors makes you a Warrior to defeat a Fat Ugly lifestyle and become victorious with a lifestyle of Looking Good, Feeling Good (LGFG). If you succeed as a Fat Warrior, you will gain your LGFG lifestyle that will be minus the FU pounds. The bonus with your new lifestyle is that you will not suffer rebound pounds.

We promise that attaining this new lifestyle will NOT be easy or quick. You will need to achieve unconditional surrender of Fat Ugly to your new Beautiful Bod. We know that you will win many battles and lose many in order to gain your permanent BB lifestyle. **You cannot lose as long as you keep fighting and don't give up. We promise you that as long as you keep fighting and improving, you will win your best Hot Bod.**

3

Your Fat Warriors Drill Sergeant

I am your Fat Warriors Drill Instructor, D.I. Don. I fight ugly fat and want to help you achieve your Beautiful Bod (BB). I will be relentless in helping you fight Fat Ugly (FU).

In the beginning, my sole motivation was to help fat people, including myself. I needed to lose my unattractive fat stomach. It was no longer a cute love handle or spare tire, it was Fat Ugly and it embarrassed me. I am becoming my personal Right Size slowly--one belt buckle hole at a time, by following the steps outlined in this book and in our first book entitled, *Don't Blame McDonald's, Did Mommy Make You Fat?* **(Order this book on our website at www.lifestyleweightexperts.com!)**

Whether you want to lose 10 pounds or 100 pounds permanently, the Fat Warriors principles will work for you.

Don is Not

Don is not a nutritionist, doctor or dietician; he is a **Lifestyle Weight Expert** and Warrior fighting fat. The Fat Warrior does not believe diets work for the long term, and is on a mission to show you a better way to reach your goal of a healthy new lifestyle and Right-Sized Bod.

Fat Warriors Must Have a War Face, Growl, and Fun!

Marines have a War Face and growl. Dogs and even puppies bare their teeth and growl, and it is scary. You must have a War Face and growl to scare fat and make it run off your hide.

Fat Warriors have a War Face, but they also have miles of smiles. They take themselves seriously, but never *too* seriously. **Our mission is to make people's lives better.** So put on your War Face, growl, and get started. Attention! Move out and read on.

How Badly Do You Want It?

The war is here and it begins with your personal battle against Fat Ugly. Fat Warriors is your ally, fighting for your life, your happiness, and your wallet. Fat Ugly has alliances with fast foods, processed foods, fat ass desserts, great tasting greasy meals, non-exercising excuses, and miracle diets, plus grandiose promises of quick and easy programs, plans, and pills. The FU alliances are all designed to make money for themselves by getting you to buy their plan, followed by coming back again and again. Get on their yo-yo cycle of losing weight and gaining it back in rebound pounds.

The Lifestyle Weight Experts' Fat Warriors program offers no miracles or instant results. We guarantee a hard-fought war that will take time. You will have weapons and a plan to win your desired and deserved lifestyle. We have no magic pill; instead you have your powerful will. You will record the food decisions you make on your ScoreCard and keep your Fatting and BB Averages, which will be discussed later in this book. We are your support, on your team, and will provide the tools to take you to your BB lifestyle. Fat Warriors are like the Marines--we are not for everyone, but if you join you just may win your most important battle for happiness and health!

It is Your Fight

It may be easier to quit now. Like any tough, great achievement, many will not be strong enough to fight and win. If you feel that you can't fight and win, then you are right. Stop now, quit now, go to the couch, and grab the chip dip. If you are Pit-Bull determined to win your war on Fat Ugly and believe you will win, then War Face on and let's go!

We will give you the tools, but make no mistake you must be the Warrior. We will war with you and be on your team, but you will and must make it *your* war and *your* fight.

CHAPTER 2

JOIN FAT WARRIORS FOR PERMANENT WEIGHT LOSS

If it were easy to be BB, nobody would be fat.

The Benefits of Being Fat Ugly
- Eat anything and all you want.
- You don't have to participate in sports, dancing, or other events.
- You don't have to reject many date offers.
- You stay warmer with your own fat coat.
- You won't have to work as hard on your career because you have less chances of being hired or offered promotional opportunities.
- You get more sympathy *(not really, people think you are fat, they just don't tell you).*
- You get to experience more diets and take more pills.
- You can participate in Width Waddlers.
- You can look forward to higher risk of heart disease, diabetes, and cancer.
- Fat floats--you can float in water.
- You can be a sumo wrestler.
- You can dominate the teeter-totter.

Join the Fat Warriors Army As a Recruit

Like the Fat Warrior, if you want to eradicate fat, you may join my Fat Warriors Army as a Recruit, advance to Private, then to Sergeant, until you achieve Fat Warrior status. You may also become a Fat Warrior D.I. That means you become a Drill Instructor and teach Recruits in boot camp to become Fat Warriors. To accomplish my dream, an Army in the *millions* will form the Fat Warriors Nation, winning Right Size freedom for the USA and beyond.

VISIT OUR WEBSITE NOW AT WWW.LIFESTYLEWEIGHTEXPERTS.COM TO FIND OUT HOW YOU CAN JOIN OUR ONLINE BOOT CAMPS!

Advancement Ranks of the Fat Warriors

Volunteer: Becomes more aware of consequences of food choices and begins to make better choices.

Recruit: Commits to learning the art of being a Fat Warrior and has purchased or read the first Fat Warriors Nation book.

Private: Trains to become a Fat Warrior. Has spent one month ScoreBooking and averaging FU and BB decisions and has shown improvement.

Sergeant:	Completes three months of ScoreBooking and averaging. BB decisions outnumber FU decisions and show positive movement toward lifestyle changes. Has read two Fat Warriors books or attended a Fat Warriors Program. Total can-do attitude.
Fat Warrior:	Pit-Bull determined mentality. Completes all books in the Fat Warriors series or attends a Fat Warriors boot camp seminar. Sustains a majority of BB decisions and demonstrates some lifestyle changes. Has taken the Fat Warriors oath and pledges to help others.
Drill Instructor:	Helps and trains others to become Fat Warriors.

The Fat Warrior Revolution

The Fat Warrior is recruiting you to join the Fat Warrior revolution and fight for your BB lifestyle. **We have a unique philosophy with a vocabulary all our own (see our Glossary of terms at the end of this book).** We invite you to join us to defeat fat. Together, let's start a revolution against Fat Ugly!

Becoming a Fat Warrior is guaranteed to be challenging, but will help lead you to a happier, healthier lifestyle. In the end, you and your Bod will feel and look victorious. You may achieve promotions and advance to Fat Warrior or even Drill Instructor status. You may then help your friends and family win their wars on fat. So, if you are ready for Fat Warriors boot camp, then be determined. Don't have onion skin.

Do have alligator hide, put on your War Face, growl, and continue marching through this book!

CHAPTER 3

SKEPTICAL? START SLIMSTYLING YOUR LIFESTYLE TODAY – JOIN FAT WARRIORS

Other programs have not worked for you so you mistrust this one.

Welcome Skeptics

Are you a doubter or disbeliever? I would be. You may ask, how can you convince me when everything else has failed? The Fat Warrior cannot convince you, but you will convince yourself. Your judgment and beliefs will convince you that you will win your goal of becoming your personal Right Size.

You Should Be Skeptical that the Lifestyle Weight Experts' Fat Warriors Program Can Help You Win a Permanent BB Lifestyle

How many of you have been on two or more diets that have failed you, and you are back wanting to lose weight again? How many vicious cycles of weight loss and rebound pounds can you mentally stand before you give up?

So if we tell you that following the Fat Warriors program could help you keep weight off permanently, you might be in disbelief. You would think the Fat Warriors concept would have to have an entirely new approach to accomplish such a miracle for you, and

11

you would be justified in that thinking. **Be confident that our approach is entirely new, and totally different, with tactics that demand permanent victory and happiness be achieved for your lifetime.** That is a far different goal than merely losing weight. Anybody can temporarily lose weight and pose for before and after pictures, only to cry later. Fat Warriors are after permanent lifestyle changes for miles of smiles.

Fat Warriors ScoreBooking Concept

The Fat Warriors concept is that **scoring food decisions is a natural self-motivator for competitive improvement. Our unique ScoreAveraging process will be explained in upcoming chapters, and if you do it, you will automatically improve YOU.** Unlike programs you have tried in the past where the plans provide the motivation and the plans are in control, as a Fat Warrior YOU will be self-motivated and in total control.

Lifestyle Weight Experts' Philosophy

How does our program differ? Why is the Fat Warriors concept different than diets? Diets are temporary fixes. They don't work because they are merely Band-Aids. Diets focus on negative goals like losing weight lightning fast instead of Right-Sizing for life. They promote unsustainable weight loss to get you (and your wallet) back again and again. **The Fat Warriors program promotes goals for a healthy lifestyle and your personal Right Size through good decisions and slow, sustainable weight loss.** The Fat Warrior did not focus on weight loss. Instead he focused on decisions that won his goal of a flat stomach. Added bonuses were lower blood pressure and lower cholesterol levels.

Fat Ugly Good News/Bad News

You, like many, have probably been on a program or involved in a support group that helped you lose weight, only to gain it back along with failure depression. That is the bad news. The good news is that you can lose weight permanently. **Fat Warriors is about you winning your war against Fat Ugly, and you can win the positive lifestyle that you OWN and desire. Instead of weight loss, envision the lifestyle you want to live.** You will make the decisions necessary to get there, and you, not a plan, will be in complete control.

Fat Warriors has no goal of weight loss, only the goal of getting you to your personal Right Size and Looking Good, Feeling Good (LGFG) lifestyle without rebound pounds. The weight loss occurs even if it is not the primary goal. Weight loss will occur slowly, but permanently, because of your decisions and new lifestyle developed by YOU.

Try Something New

It is time to try something totally different because your brain tells you it will work. Instead of a spokesperson or testimonials selling you on their plans, your brain cells and your self-motivation say let's do it! Your Bod and heart agree. You expect promises of easy and fast weight loss, but this concept is slow and challenging!

Overhaul Your Current Mindset!

Understand that you are not overweight. **You are at your perfect weight for the lifestyle and decisions you are currently making.**

Overhaul your mindset and you can change the only two things that will lead to your Beautiful Bod and healthy lifestyle: decisions and lifestyle changes.

It's time to clear your mind and eliminate preconceived opinions. First, lose the attitude of *I can't*, and change it to *I can. I can do it, I can do more,*

13

I can do more than I think. Lose anything that has not worked for you if your Beautiful Bod is imprisoned in layers of Fat Ugly. Your BB is about to fight. Toss out all things that have failed--scales, quick and easy diet plans, and pills. Excuses must go too--take the next step. Whenever you need more war power, revisit your mirror. It will tell you that you must, can, and will win and defeat Fat Ugly. War Face on!

> ## *Change your mind before you shortchange your Bod.*

"What If" Game

What if the Lifestyle Weight Experts' Fat Warriors Program just might work for you? What if...Would you open your mind to give it a try? Think about it, what have you got to lose except misery? With the Fat Warriors program, there is little cost in time or money. What if your judgment, not trickery or before and after pictures, convinced you that this just might be what you've been waiting for? If that is the case, you are ready to fight your Fat Ugly war. You will win permanent lifestyle victory if...YOU WILL ASSUME VALUE AND RESERVE JUDGMENT. If you don't try, you will never know and possibly remain fat forever.

CHAPTER 4

ABANDON FAT SHIP: WHY DIETS AND CALORIE COUNTING FAILED **YOU**

Are You a DietHolic? Take the Test
- Have you been on more than three diet plans, only to rebound and start your next miracle diet?

- Have you tried to lose weight with each program, but lost only wallet and can-do confidence?

- Do before and after pictures help persuade you to buy diet pills, plans, magic shakes or fat burners?

- Do you spend more time counting calories than counting on yourself?

- Do you look down at scales more than looking up at life and fun?

Kick the DietHolic addiction's ass, save your money and look like a honey! Go to www.lifestyleweightexperts.com.

A Diet by Any Other Name …

The Lifestyle Weight Experts' Fat Warriors Program has been preaching the only success diets have is a high failure rate and permanent wallet loss. Many diet program companies have spent much money removing the word "diet" from their advertisements because they experience too much rebound Fat Ugly. Why is that? Is it because the Lifestyle Weight Experts Team has been drumming that dieters experience more rebound pounds than weight loss? Diets quickly remove the diet name from literature, but the contents of their programs remain the same. If the content is the same, your results will be … da same? How do you spot a diet when the diet name has been removed? Get clues, Sherlock!

Detective Clues to Spot Disguised Diets: What Sherlock diet clues can you send to lifestyleweightexperts.com?

- Responsibility and money are taken from you and given to the plan.
- They motivate by before and after pictures (grab wallet and run).
- They use celebrities to convince you to try their plan.
- Their success is determined by you losing weight while on the plan.
- They have you weighing daily and measuring success by weight loss in days.
- They have you counting calories daily or pointing out points.
- You lose permanent wallet and gain depression.
- You have regained weight after the plan and are now repeating the plan.

> *Diets are more interested in their bottom line than your bottom. Bottom out on them.*

Permanent Money Loss and Temporary Weight Loss

If you have felt the emotional and physical pains of Fat Ugly, then it is likely that you have tried every diet, pill, blaster, dynamite powder, and machine that is available, only to be back again and again after rebound pounds appear. Rebounding is great for basketball, but not for weight gain.

If this is your story, then it is time for a new paradigm and something that will work. Get off the couch and put on your War Face. **The more times you use fad diets, the more they make money while you lose your money and your will. Become a Fat Warrior and trim fad diets' profit lines as you trim your waistline. You will be TrimStyling in your new Hot Bod!**

Diet Pills Are for People Who Believe There Is an Easy Cure in a Pill

Lose 100 pounds in 100 days, take this pill and lose weight, guaranteed! Get your first bottle of fat spanker pills free and then only pay for the next 40 bottles! Guaranteed to work or return for full refund! Companies that sell these products know that only a small percentage of people will send them back for a refund. Most people would not go to the trouble or embarrassment of packaging the magic pills and returning them.

Taking diet pills shows that you can't cut it and are delegating your fat problem to a pharmaceutical company, whose main mission is to keep you buying

17

more pills. Pills only give you false hope and an excuse to treat eat.

**Count out counting calories for permanent
lifestyle change.**

What Does Calorie Counting Have to Do With Weight Loss?

The fact is calorie counting did not make you fat, and it will not help you win your personal Right Size. You have probably counted cals before and failed, and so counting them is neither the cause nor the solution. You must understand this to escape the fat cycle.

It helps you know that eating pie topped with ice cream has a lot of calories. Calorie counting may improve your math skills, but it becomes a detractor and causes you to lose focus on the one thing that can win your wonderful lifestyle permanently: decisions.

If you know the difference between a brownie and an apple, then bite into the apple. No calorie counting needed, unless you eat a bushel of apples at a sitting. In that case, apple deleting will occur as the fiber content rises.

Everybody is afraid to say anything for fear of offending. –Dean Ottati, The Runner and the Path

---

Any Amount of FU Pain Is Devastating

How many of you right now admit that you have a weight problem and are 6 ounces or more overweight? How about 16 ounces or more? (That is one pound for you non-math majors.)

You are probably asking yourself, "Is he going to ask how many of us are 50 pounds, 100 pounds, or more overweight?" People don't like Fat Warriors to ask the big poundage questions because it might embarrass fat people. However, Fat Warriors philosophy is that it is helpful to admit it and feel the embarrassment. If it does not embarrass you, then you will likely never lose weight and you will soon see why.

If you are comfortable with your current FatStyle, then you will have no motivation for change. The more uncomfortable you are with it, the better your chances of gaining back your personal Right Size. TrimStyle instead of FatStyle!

More Than 100 Pounds? May Need Medical Attention

The amazing thing is that people who want to lose 10 pounds struggle with the emotions of not looking good, feeling mentally and physically unfit, and experience much of the same pains as people who are 100 pounds overweight.

The people who are beyond 100 pounds overweight may be experiencing more serious medical and/or emotional problems that may be far more devastating than those trying to take off fewer pounds.

No matter how many pounds a person is overweight, the emotional consequences are painful, but those of you 100 or more pounds overweight should seek close monitoring of weight loss by a physician.

> *You might have to hit rock bottom to change the*
> *size of your bottom.*

Change Your Mind and Your Goal

Start with a fresh mind. **Your goal should not be weight loss, but gaining your personal Right Size for life.**

You are the difference. You are the plan. You own the consequences and the benefits. The entire process is directed, planned and controlled by you. It will never leave you and you own it for life.

CHAPTER 5

FAT UGLY ANALYSIS: HELP FOR **YOU**

Things that matter most must never be at the mercy of things that matter least. -
Goethe

Are You Fat? Take the Test

- I find it fun____ / embarrassing____ to shop for clothes.
- People do____ / do not____ notice what I order at restaurants.
- I love____ / hate____ to walk out in public and be seen by people.
- My significant other is proud____ / embarrassed____ to be seen with me.
- I love____ / hate____ my mirror.
- I think I look great____ / awful____.
- Thoughts about my Bod boost____ / sink____ my self-esteem.
- True____ or False____: I spend more time worrying about my Bod shape than shaping up.
- True____ or False____: I must select my chair by its strength or width rather than comfort.
- True____ or False____: My partner will turn off the lights.

Your Story of How You Became Fat Ugly

If you are fat, to understand your progression to a Fat Ugly lifestyle you need to define the approximate time you started doing things differently. For example, when you started eating more fat foods, processed foods, desserts, ice cream, going to Fataurants, or drinking soda pop. These factors started adding on fat gradually. **It was a slow lifestyle change, until one day you realized that you had lost control. You looked in the mirror and Fat Ugly looked back at you.**

Pinpointing when and what changes occurred is important to understanding what caused you to gradually plump up. How long did it take you to totally lose control? Knowing the answers to these questions will help you **understand why you gained fat, and that is the secret to knowing how to reverse it.**

If you understand the changes, only then can you be on your way back to your LGFG lifestyle. It will mean a Fat Ugly war, but you will understand why you can win because you will understand why you lost.

Ask Yourself:

- What causes me to be fat?
- How long have I been fat?
- How did I get to be so big? How many days or years did it take to become Fat Ugly?
- Am I still building myself bigger?
- What will I look like five years from today if I continue this?
- Am I still feeling sorry for myself?
- What is the cost to my health?
- What are my doctor's comments?
- How do I feel after walking up stairs?
- What has it cost me in the job market in dollars over the years?
- How much does it cost in embarrassment?
- What is the toll on my love life?

- How much pleasure do I get from buying fat clothes?
- How many pains can I name that come from my fat?
- Do I hang with fat people, and do they make me feel more comfortable by being with them?
- How do I look in a bathing suit?
- When will I take my Best Bod back and gain my new lifestyle?

Journal It

Begin your self-revealing journey by writing three letters to yourself. The first letter should describe your feelings about being Fat Ugly now. The second should relay your feelings about how you will feel if you continue your current lifestyle and nothing changes. The third letter should be about the life that you visualize or dream of having with your LGFG lifestyle. Keep a journal about your struggles and triumphs. Refer to it often, and use it for inspiration to never give up.

CHAPTER 6

SELL YOURSELF:
YOU CAN CAN THE FATCAN

Cognitive Dissonance: The Difference Between What You Have and What You *Want*!

Cognitive dissonance is the difference between what you have and what you want. Mirror yourself right now for your cognitive dissonance. *While you look like this now, do you want to look like this for 10, 20, or 30 years? When you think about this, it is a horrifying life sentence.* People act for change only when they reach a pain threshold of cognitive dissonance. **If you experience the pain of cognitive dissonance, you can start making winning decisions right now and win one decision at a time for your lifetime of more smiles, happiness, and health.**

Magic Moment

Wow, this Fat Ugly cognitive dissonance is sad and an emotionally depressing evaluation when you are fat. On the other hand, you can see clearly what you want and turn it into your magic moment. **Your magic moment is when you decide that you want to become your personal Right Size so bad that you will fight and make the BB decisions necessary to attain it.** Know your cognitive dissonance, feel the pain, and pain will motivate you to change to win the lifestyle you deserve.

Cognitive dissonance is the difference between what you have and what you want. **Ask yourself, "What is my cognitive dissonance?"**

24

Cognitive Dissonance Examples:
- Fat Ugly unattractiveness vs. Beautiful Bod attractiveness
- The Bod you see vs. the Bod you want, plus the joys and health it will bring
- Emotional embarrassment with your FU Bod vs. the proud feeling you can achieve with your Beautiful Bod
- The unhealthy dangers of Fat Ugly vs. the healthy lifestyle benefits of a Beautiful Bod
- Pills vs. treadmill
- Dating down Fat Ugly vs. dating up Beautiful Bod
- Avoiding vs. participating
- Fat clothes vs. cool clothes
- Fat Ugly lifestyle vs. Looking Good, Feeling Good (LGFG) lifestyle

---

Think of your cognitive dissonance examples and list your Top 10. Share them on www.lifestyleweightexperts.com!

Cognitive Dissonance: Paying the Price
- You are tired of your old car that looks bad and breaks down; you pay the price and get a newer car.
- My personal one. I felt the emotional and physical pains of smoking; I paid the price and finally made it to permanent quit and non-smoking lifestyle change.

- You dislike your hairstyle; you pay the price for a new style and feel the joy of people complimenting you on your new do.
- You are tired and feel out of shape; you pay the price and feel the exhilaration and new-found energy that exercise brings.

Create your cognitive dissonance, the difference in what you have and what you want. What is the price, if any, you are willing to pay? **You must feel and visualize the pain to help give you the strength and discipline to win.**

Go sit in Fataurants, all-you-can-eat stuffets, clothing stores, anywhere. Watch what the waddlers order. Watch them eat, walk, climb stairs, not participate, be embarrassed. Watch them shop for clothes; look at their clothes. Look at them, and imagine that is you now and forever if you do not pay the price to change.

You must see your future pain before you can change.

Cognitive Dissonance: The Pain Causes Change

Focus on what you want and insist on getting it. You don't want to lose weight; you really want to look great and feel great! That is a more positive goal worth fighting for. Imagine you new looks, health, and smoking Bod Hot lifestyle.

Smoking Out My Love Life

I was addicted to cigarettes, and had proof of my unhealthy lifestyle with stinky breath and bad lungs. I went through 25 years of quitting and relapsing. However, I knew my cognitive dissonance. I wanted the benefits of a smoke-free lifestyle so much that I did not give up. I believed that I could do it, but then I realized that it was not as hard as fighting lung cancer and not being able to date the non-smoking, hot cuties.

I would not date smoking women, and non-smoking women would not date me. My love life was to be absent of the opposites as long as I smoked. Not having the opportunity for the good-breath women was a bigger pain than giving up smoking.

The right motivation came along, and I am thankful it was a cute woman and not a lung surgeon. After about a year, the decision not to smoke had become a lifestyle change. I became a nonsmoker who would never smoke again.

Thinking, thoughts, and decisions drove me into that smoking habit and victim mentality. My cognitive dissonance drove my thoughts about the pains of smoking versus the pains of quitting, which drove my decisions that led to my lifestyle change to a nonsmoker. Now that I am not a smoker, I think smokers just lack discipline. Easy to say now! What do people say about fat people?

I have not smoked in years and don't miss it one bit. I don't miss the cigarette breath, shortness of breath, and having to go to the North Pole to have a smoke.

Incidentally, just like fat people, smokers say they have tried everything and just can't quit. The fact is, if both groups keep fighting they'll eventually win. **Persistence is key!**

The only thing worse than being a smoker is being a fat smoker. You have to be blind and dumb not to see the parallel between being fat and smoking. Both are embarrassing, depressing, costly, ugly, and can kill you. The question must be answered, are they worth the price?

CHAPTER 7

SCORING, SEX, LOVE, HEALTH, WEALTH POWERS – WIN THIN MOTIVATION!

An intelligent plan is the first step to success. The man who plans knows where he is going, knows what progress he is making, and has a pretty good idea when he will arrive. -Basil Walsh

ScoreBooking: Path to Permanent Right-Sized Lifestyle

Do you want to lose wide hide permanently? Keep score and average! Need powerized self-motivation for making decisions to exercise and eat right? Then keep your score and average!   Need the self-discipline to make decisions not to eat candy bars or other Fuglies? Then ScoreBook and average!

Weight loss that is not permanent becomes rebound fat. The fact is that losing weight is easy, but keeping it off is not. Achieving and maintaining your personal Right Size requires self-motivation and self-discipline. **Making great decisions and ScoreBooking & averaging means less jiggle in your wiggle.**

With Fat Warriors you will keep your decisions score. We will show you how to get started with our easy-to-use ScoreBooking technique.

28

Your Triple Crown Jewels of Life

Just as in other areas of life, keeping track of your decisions on a daily basis will naturally provide you with relentless and powerful self-motivation to Right Size. Recording decisions is easy fun. You will see that scoring points is the way to discover a treasure chest filled with the jewels of your new envisioned lifestyle. You will be aware of every decision affecting your BB and FU Averages, and that will have you:

- Looking your best
- Feeling your best
- Creating euphoric feelings
- Averaging and seeing the results on your ScoreCard, your mind, and in the mirror
- Attaining your best health
- Attaining optimum income
- Enjoying your best life possible

Win Your Right Size by Keeping Score and Averaging

Have you ever bowled a 300 game, a 200 game, or how about your first 100 game? Have you ever broken par or broken 100 in golf? Have you ever played baseball, tennis, or any game? Have you ever owned a business? **These activities involve keeping score, which optimizes the self-motivation and discipline to improve or win.** Without scoring and averages, there would be no winners, losers, tournaments, games, or championships.

Without records and scorekeeping, few athletes would be motivated to improve. Without scoring there would be no records, and we know that records are made to be broken--just like your rebound fat cycle.

It is a key concept that without keeping sports scores, few would play, fewer would watch, and nobody would win! You will see why ScoreBooking & Averaging provides powerful self-motivation to win your permanent Best Bod.

Scoring & Averaging Is Easy and Necessary for Winning Your BB

- How do you know if your golf game is improving? *You look at your score card.*
- How do we know who won the football game or the Super Bowl? *By looking at the final score.*
- What is the basis for betting games? *Betting on the score.*
- What do you see in a bowling alley? *Big, electric projecting scoreboards.*
- How is a baseball game won? *By the number of runs scored.*
- How do athletes know if they are improving? *In baseball, it is the batting average; in bowling, it is averaging the number of pins per game; in football, it is the average per carry.*

In the game of golf, you want a low score to win. In bowling, you want a high score and consequent high average. When you record that great game, it is on the card for show and tell for the world to see. Businesses keep score on an income statement. When you record your first profits, big smiles are generated as people look at and share the positive scored results. Keeping score in business is so important that it has its own name: the *bottom line*. **The point is that winning usually involves the keeping of scores and averaging to demonstrate success or progress.**

People even score in the dating game. Baseball players run around the bases and constantly check improvements in their batting average. Scoring and averaging can signal success and is necessary for motivation, fun, and improvement. ScoreBooking puts the excitement and fun in the game, and leads to your personal Right Size.

You can't have a motivated bowler, ball player or golfer who does not keep score and average. As a Fat Warrior, you will keep score on your personal ScoreCard, which will strengthen your resolve to make BB decisions. Read on, and we will show you how. You will see that ScoreAveraging takes only minutes to do, but pays off with your permanent Best Bod lifestyle.

> *Pain Week is a week to realize that what you have become affects your core of Body, Mind, and Spirit.*

Pain Week and Fabits

Your first week as a Fat Warriors recruit is Pain Week. This week is your starting line of ScoreBooking and reflecting on your weaknesses and Fat habits ("Fabits"). It is your week of recognizing why and how your Bod grew to FU. **It is not a week of guilt, but a week of understanding.** It is a week to experience the pains of owning Fat Ugly. It is time to determine how FU affects your feelings, mood, social life, participation, career, health, wealth, and self-esteem.

A Week to Peek

Pain Week is seven days of opening your eyes to understand the effects of your Fat Ugly lifestyle. What you normally eat, do, drink, and think is likely what began your FU journey a long time ago. During Pain Week, you will note on your ScoreCard what you eat, the amount you consume, and the amount of exercise (or lack of it). Very important is to think about what you think about! Example: If you think enough about not eating the banana split, it will soon split your lips as you eat it. What you think about tends to happen as the Law of Fattraction rules.

Pain week is about feeling the pain, identifying and understanding what causes your current decisions that keep you imprisoned in Fat Ugly. When it is over, you have completed the first step to becoming a Private in the Fat Warriors Army. Pain Week provides the self-motivation to win a BB permanent lifestyle. Any program that does not focus on paying the price for a new and permanent lifestyle results in devastating rebound pounds.

P.S. Those who skip Pain Week and just start into recording based on memory of their history (routine) may do so without being sent to the Fat Brig. But you must really understand all of your pains both mental and physical.

Lies Have More Hidden Calories than a Chocolate Cake

Truth is essential for accurate ScoreAveraging. No deceit, hiding, or lying about the chocolate lying in your purse. Stashing fat snacks in drawers, under pillows, and other favorite hiding places is sabotaging your success. If you are doing it, why are you doing it, and who are you hiding it from? Bring them out, let everybody, including you, see them. Feel the shame, and that pain may cause you not to do it.

Benchmark Musts for Gaining Your Personal Right Size

Benchmarks are a must for Right-Sizing. To create benchmarks, you must begin scoring and averaging for improvement.

Grades cause people to study, gold medals cause people to train, money causes people to work, and bonuses cause people to out-perform goals. Performance, scores and averages are kept, recorded, compared, and supply needed self-motivation.

If you are determined to win your war, you must average and compare your decision benchmarks. Do that and you will start making more positive decisions, which will turn your dream size into permanent reality. Recording and comparing averages is mandatory to show your progress and optimize your chance of success. **Do you want your new lifestyle? Then you must score and average. Read on, we will show you how ScoreAveraging works!**

CHAPTER 8

WHY SCORING +
CALCULATING FATTING
AVERAGE =
PERMANENT WEIGHT LOSS

The Lifestyle Weight Experts' ScoreCard may alone cause more permanent success than all fad diets, miracle pills or other programs combined.

ScoreBooking: The Powerful Secret to Your Permanent Right Size

Daily and weekly food decisions can be recorded in a small notebook or on the official Lifestyle Weight Experts' ScoreCard that you can download from our website at www.lifestyleweightexperts.com. We will provide you with suggested scoring methods and show you how to calculate your Beautiful Bod (BB) Average and your Fat Ugly (FU or Fatting) Average.

- Carry your **ScoreCard** with you at all times for convenient decisions recordings. I suggest scoring once daily.

- Use your **ScoreCard** to plan, record and optimize decreasing your percentage of FUs while increasing BB decisions. See the improvements in averages.

- Once a day record your FU and BB decisions on your **ScoreCard**. It is easy and quick, and you can do this in less than one minute. That's right, it takes less than 60 seconds a day to **ScoreBook** your decisions! Will you pay the price for increasing your success by 100 percent?

- Did you miss a day or two of recording your decisions? No problem! Just start **ScoreBooking** again. Missing is expected and not important, as long as you start recording and averaging again.

- We will explain how to calculate your BB Average and Fatting Average on your **ScoreCard** to optimize your natural competitive spirit to make more BB decisions. You can calculate your weekly average in two minutes or less.

- Your **ScoreCard** will help you achieve your goals for the LGFG Promised Land. **ScoreBooking** will leave you feeling proud and healthy when you have attained the level of behavior that is sustainable for you.

- **ScoreBooking** is not an option, but a must for optimum lifetime results to eliminate rebound pounds. **ScoreBooking** provides encouraging self-motivation and discipline for a sustainable win of your personal Right Size.

Player, Coach and Referee!

ScoreBooking can be a fun and challenging game. You are the player, coach, judge, and referee. You decide the FUs and BBs. This is your tool to cause a change in decisions to help you reach your goal. When you reduce your FUs, you will automatically

35

increase BBs. As your BB decisions increase, your weight will slowly decrease.

FU Decision ("Fugly"): A Fat Ugly decision, like downing a Twinkie instead of grapes or deciding not to exercise. Measure decisions not food!

BB Decision ("BB"): A Beautiful Bod decision, like eating an apple instead of a brownie. Not having the glass of wine at night is a BB for me.

Keeping Score with Your ScoreCard

If you have ever kept score in baseball or card games like bridge, you know scoring principles. The way Fat Warriors keep score is simple, and easier to learn and use.

<u>Suggested Notations for ScoreBooking:</u>

FU	Fugly--used for Fat decisions or Fat foods
BB	BB--used for good decisions
B	Breakfast
L	Lunch
D	Dinner
S	Snack
d	Drink--alcohol or sugar-based beverages
E	Exercise

Here are some decision examples that will show you how easy it is to keep score:

- **Foods you select**: For example, a brownie is an FU and an apple is a BB.
- **Portion sizes**: A portion size that is too large or too small is an FU, and a Right-Sized portion is a BB.

- **Bad decisions**: Starving or skipping a meal like breakfast is an FU.
- **Having a healthy breakfast**: Oatmeal, banana, whole-wheat toast and juice = BBs.
- **A not-so-healthy breakfast**: A jelly roll is an FU.
- **Daily exercise**: This is a BB, and an extra-long session might be two BBs.
- **No daily exercise**: Always an FU unless a rest day.
- **Indulging a Fat Ugly habit ("Fabit")**: For example, raiding the fridge at 11:00 p.m. is an FU.
- **Giving up a bad Fabit**: Not grazing on snacks while watching TV is a BB.
- **Having sex**: At least one BB, sometimes two. Remember, this should be fun!
- **A 20-minute pause** to prevent over-portion eating (a/k/a the 20-Minute Rule) = 2 BBs (one for smaller portion and one for not eating large).
- **Participating in BB behavior** that will fit you into your jeans, such as a decision to eliminate a bad Fabit like eating potato chips every day = BB.
- **Participating in FU behavior** that perpetuates your Fat Ugly lifestyle, like continuing to drink sugar-laden beverages = FU.
- **Selecting Fugly friends** for comfort eating = FU.
- **Selecting BB friends** for role models = BB.
- **ScoreBooking** daily = BB, Averaging weekly = BB.
- **Selecting doors that open into establishments like all-you-can-eat stuffets, dreamy queens and doughnut shops** = 1-3 FUs just for entering.
- **Pre-planning your day** to choose more BBs than Fuglies = BB, and sticking to it is another BB.

- **Grocery store list** pre-planned for a healthy cart and sticking to it at the store = 1-5 BBs for a great decision cart!

First, prioritize a few key Fuglies and Fabits that you want to change. In fact, you may want to list your Fuglies and Fabits. Make these your priority decisions for starters. It is best to work in baby steps, only changing 1-3 Fabits at a time. Examples:

- Not routinely eating potato chips or fries.

- Not eating after 7:30 p.m.

- Practicing Right-Sized portions and the 20-Minute Rule, which means don't eat until stuffed. Instead, stop when comfortable, wait 20 minutes, and see if you still want more.

ScoreBooking makes you more aware of big decisions, allowing you to wear smaller clothes.

Measuring Decisions, Not Food or Calories, Etc.

BB and FU decisions are what you will be measuring. You will not be measuring bad foods, exercise, portions or calories. You may customize your decisions to what makes the most sense for you. My best example is that I used to have a ritual of snacking every night before bed. Now any time I make the decision to skip this ritual Fabit, I reward myself with a BB on my ScoreCard. By making this BB decision, those nocturnal calories and guilt do not lie in my stomach and weigh on my mind, disturbing my digestion and sleep. If I decide to have a late-night snack, it goes onto my ScoreCard as a Fugly and lies with me all night long.

This means recording decisions like eating a large portion or more than one portion as an FU, and a properly sized, healthy portion as a BB. **Eating a portion that's too small or nothing at all records as an FU, because too little or deprivation is neither healthy nor sustainable.** Similarly, the decision to exercise is a BB, and no exercise is a Fugly unless it is a rest day. A movie tub of FatCorn is an FU; the decision to not have it is a BB, while diet soda may be a BB depending on whether or not you believe in zero-calorie sweeteners. Alcohol drinks are Fuglies (yes, even beer and wine), so if you drink, cut it down. Each drink you skip is a BB. Each drink you have is an FU.

Say Yes to Nots
"Nots" can be BBs: not eating food after the evening meal, not snacking while watching TV, not eating high-calorie rich desserts, not eating high-fat foods, not pigging out at work, not downing bags of chips, and more. Not eating until stuffed and practicing the 20-Minute Rule is a great BB.

You will become aware of your BBs and Fuglies and see that they reach much further than just food. **Daring to be aware and thinking about your decisions and consequences will help you make better decisions for your permanent Right-Size goal.**

Have a Plan
You will occasionally make FU decisions, and starting out you may make many. Your goal will be to improve steadily. ScoreBook them, be honest. Feel good being aware and slowly improving.

There is logic for setting an attainable, realistic goal for success. If you set the goal and attain it, no matter how small the improvement, give yourself 5 extra BBs!

Because the decision to plan to achieve is in itself a BB. Attaining it is another BB. It is the super bonus for sticking with your plan and having the discipline to make the decisions and improve your average. However, it may take time to make this improvement because no one is perfect. Just keep fighting for your lifestyle.

ScoreBooking decisions is key to your Right-Sizing victory. Anyone can do it. **You will understand why scoring is crucial to your self-motivation and discipline for winning your LGFG lifestyle. You will also calculate your BB and Fatting Averages, which will be discussed in the next chapter.**

Real ScoreCard Examples of the Fat Warrior

I use the same abbreviations provided above on my ScoreCard: **B**=Breakfast, **L**=Lunch, **D**=Dinner, **S**=Snack, **E**=Exercise, **d**=drink. **BB**=Beautiful Bod, **FU**=**Fat Ugly**. I also make small letter notations beside my Fuglies and BBs to help me remember what contributed to each decision. You may choose to do this, too, so you can see what led to your BB and FU decisions. You will want to develop your own scoring codes.

>   **B**: BB, BB   (oatmeal with banana & berries, and whole-wheat toast)
>   **E**: BB (one BB for each 30 minutes of exercise)
>   **S**: BB-a (apple & raw almonds)
>   **L**: BB, FU (grilled chicken breast, and potato salad with mayonnaise)
>   **D**: BB, FU-d, FU-d (proper portion of grilled fish with two glasses of wine)

Pain in the Butt?

ScoreBooking should be almost painless and fun when you see the improvements. It takes no more than a minute or two per day. At the end of the day or at any time, write down your decisions for the day or the last couple of days. For example, once daily I record my scores on my ScoreCard. I do this at whatever time is most convenient. One evening I might take out my ScoreCard and record my decisions for yesterday and today. Sometimes I do it in the morning as I recall what decisions I made yesterday, but mostly I do it in the evening. **This is a 60-second investment in my Best Bod and it will give you your Best Bod if you do it!**

Turn Up the Music, Step on the ScoreBooking Accelerator, and Enjoy the Drive

By ScoreBooking, soon you will be breaking Fabits and the pain of change will be in your rear view mirror. Winning on your ScoreCard is like driving your car in sunshine with the music up and sunroof open.

Think of driving your sleek Hot Bod down to the corner of Euphoria and Hottie Drive. If you are willing to invest 60 seconds a day in your Bod, this simple investment only requires carrying a small notebook in your pocket or purse for recording your FUs and BBs. The mileage you get from your Hot Bod can be fantastic, depending on the fuel you put into the tank. Fat Warriors know that you are in charge of your decisions and your Bod.

Your figure will look like the figures on your ScoreCard.

The powerful benefits of ScoreBooking will make you stronger, happier, and more positive

41

about yourself as you win back your Right-Sized Bod. Each BB decision will be a little badge of victory. You will eventually have strings of BBs, bringing feelings of achievement and lifestyle-changing victory.

Some say it works best to break ScoreBooking into small chunks, so do one week of ScoreBooking to experience it and see the progress it helps deliver. Your ScoreCard will be quite revealing of your Right-Sizing decisions and begin to reveal your best Hot Bod. **You'll get an idea of how many Fabits you have, when they happen, and when you change them. Take one baby step, breaking one Fabit at a time, and commit to ScoreBooking for one month** *now*! **It is best to baby-step, only trying to change three Fabits or less at a time. Win three and on to the next three!**

ScoreBooking for Success

Your ScoreCard will clearly show your losses and wins. You do not become a great baseball player overnight; you will always have some strikeouts and home runs. The idea is to improve as a hitter. The fact is that without scoring, you will be able to see your progression toward your personal Right Size.

"Slow but steady" is a part of the process, as it is merely one good decision after another repeated over time to get to your Beautiful Bod. Gradually, Fabits will start disappearing and no longer dominate your thoughts.

Let Your ScoreCard Be a Conversation Piece With Friends and Family

It is a natural human trait that you will keep trying to improve your decision making if you keep track of your decisions on your ScoreCard. Just as sure as you got Fat Ugly, this will help you win your Beautiful Bod. Brag about your BB decisions to your friends and family.   FUs and BBs become a great conversation topic and source of encouragement.

You can have fun competing with yourself or with friends for improvement.   This is a true game of life, and you can win your dream lifestyle. Wow, how fun to play the Fat Warriors scoring game and what cool rewards. You may be in the Hall of Shame today and in the Hall of Fame next year!

CHAPTER 9

EASILY CALCULATE YOUR FATTING AVERAGE & BB AVERAGE

Nobody succeeds beyond his or her wildest expectations unless he or she begins with some wild expectations. –
Ralph Charell

Your BB Average vs. Your Fatting Average

We know how important the batting average is to baseball players. The same importance applies to Fat Warriors performance. **Instead of a batting average, in Fat Warriors you will have a Beautiful Bod or Best Bod Average ("BB Average") and a Fat Ugly Average ("Fatting Average").**

Easy to Calculate Your BB and FU Averages!

To calculate your **BB Average**, take your total number of BB decisions and divide by your total number of BB and FU decisions.

To calculate your **Fatting Average**, take your total number of FU decisions and divide by your total number of BB and FU decisions.

So for example, out of 10 decisions made this day, nine of them were Fat Ugly, and one was Beautiful Bod.

44

> *Nine FU decisions out of a total of 10 FU plus BB decisions = Fatting Average of 900.*
> *One BB decision out of a total of 10 FU & one BB decisions = BB Average of 100.*

Keep in mind that the total of your Fatting Average + BB Average will always be 1,000 or 1.0.

Example: BB Average
Seven BB decisions divided by 10 total BB and FU decisions equals a BB Average of 700 (7 BBs / 10 total decisions = .700).

Example: Fatting Average
Three FU decisions divided by 10 total BB and FU decisions equals a Fatting Average of 300 (3 FUs / 10 total decisions = .300).

Remember, the sum of your BB Average and Fatting Average will always be 1000 or 1.0.

Great News!
If you are currently Fat Ugly, then your Fatting Average will be high and your BB Average will be low. The great news is that you only need to start making small improvements slowly to win more BBs and begin regaining your permanent Right Size, complete with a healthy new lifestyle. **You will have grins instead of chins.**

You only need total focus on hitting more BBs and swinging at fewer FUs. At first, like learning to hit a ball, it will be difficult, but it will become easier because you will learn to be a better decision hitter.

Repeated BB decisions are the only thing that will change your Fat Ugly lifestyle to a permanent healthy, happy lifestyle. Diets have failed you at accomplishing this, but decisions won't. Calorie counting has failed you, but averaging won't.

More Fun Examples of BB and Fatting Averages

Tally your FUs and BBs at the end of the day and end of the week, and calculate for Fatting Average and BB Average once a week. These FUN averages will propel you to the best decisions and your Right-Size lifestyle. It is a walk-off winner for you!

Pretend you are now an experienced Fat Warrior. You have your eye on the BB decision ball and you record 100 decisions in one week--90 BBs and 10 FUs.

Again, for your **BB Average**, take your total number of BB decisions and divide them by your total number of BB and FU decisions:

> ➤ *90 BB decisions divided by 100 total BB and FU decisions equals a BB Average of 900 (90 BB / 100 total decisions = .900).*

For your **Fatting Average**, take your total number of FU decisions and divide them by your total number of BB and FU decisions.

> ➤ *10 FU decisions divided by 100 total BB and FU decisions equals a Fatting Average of 100 (10 FUs / 100 total decisions = .100).*

Your Fatting Average dropped from 900 to 100 and your BB Average rose from 100 to 900. See how recording and calculating your averages lets you track the dramatic improvement toward your Looking Good, Feeling Good lifestyle?

ScoreAveraging decisions is the key to self-motivation and discipline to make your dream lifestyle become reality, permanently. ScoreBook it! See our website www.lifestyleweightexperts.com.

Remember, You Are Scoring and Averaging Decisions, Not Food

Now you know the importance of keeping your score and averages for winning your Beautiful Bod. Whether you decide on the apple for a snack (BB), or the brownie (FU), score the decision, not the food. **Your lifestyle change will come from repeating positive decisions. That leap from decisions to lifestyle change will lead you to the accomplishments you desire.** Think of it as your Self-Super Bowl. When you get there, your pantry will be filled with healthy foods instead of pudding. You will be TrimStyling and feeling terrific. You will laugh at pudding and whip whipped cream.

If baseball, golf, football, ice skating, business, music, and even the weather measures performance, then why not you? By averaging, you can gain permanent life rewards of enrichments instead of pounds.

CHAPTER 10

DECISIONS ARE FAT
BLASTERS AND
BELLY FASCINATORS

Your mission as Fat Warriors is to seek and destroy Fuglies with more BB decisions every day.
The decisions are the keys to winning battles, and winning battles is the key to driving your new Hot Bod around town.

Which Is Most Important, Weight Loss or Positive Decisions Control?

Fat Warriors know that it is important to look at food as *decisions*. Decisions are your secret weapons that will kick fat's ass. FU decisions have been making you fat. Really? It's just decisions that are making me fat, not food? Yep. You thought it was the candy bars, doughnuts, ice cream, or MochaChocaLattes. Nope, it was the decisions that put them within reach and then into your mouth.

Listen to your mind instead of your tongue.

Your MIND Is in Charge

Decisions are from the mind, and you are directly responsible for your Fat Ugly or BB decisions. Your success has everything to do with what is inside your mind and not some company's outside program. It is all attributed to you, not a diet, magical plan or miracle pill. It is within you and it is a result of your self-empowerment and winning BB decisions. For once you are in charge, in control, and you confidently know it.

Train Your Brain

The only successful weight system is free and is hosted by your skull. It resides inside your head and is called your brain. It makes your decisions, good and bad. You are the in-charge programmer of your brain. You will it and control it. If you keep making the right decisions, your brain will program itself to think that way.

Train your brain to want a Beautiful Bod and keep making BB decisions. **Each BB decision will be a little bit easier until one day your brain will become brainwashed by good decisions until they become normal behavior. At this point, you have a *lifestyle* change.**

No Starving. Starving yourself is sabotage and accomplishes only one thing: it makes you hungry and causes pig outs. Starving and going hungry have no place in being a Fat Warrior. Make the decision to eat more nutritiously and never starve!

Morning Reveille

Start in the morning with a chant to yourself. Plan and envision the Beautiful Bod decisions you will make that day and every benefit of your new BB lifestyle. Jump inside that dream, live it and feel it. Take your dream lifestyle with you everywhere. Do not hit the scale or it will hit you with thoughts of weight loss. Instead, clean your weapons, lock and load for BB decisions and move out with positive steps. Patrol all day and play Taps at night.

Fat Ugly IQ Test: Which Decisions Are Best for Beautiful Bod?

- Ice cream vs. frozen yogurt
- Brownie vs. apple
- White flour bread vs. multi-grain bread
- Regular Coke vs. Diet Coke
- Candy wrapper vs. food label
- Starbucks Fat Dome with whipped cream and sprinkles vs. regular coffee or iced tea
- McDonald's loaded cheese pounder with fat fries vs. McD's grilled chicken salad
- Snacking while TV-ing it, watching fat grow on you vs. walking, jogging or biking for 20 minutes
- Peanut butter and jelly sandwich vs. peanut butter only on an open-face sandwich
- Sugar-laden soft drinks vs. diet soda/water
- Getting up at night and raiding the fridge vs. not eating after 7:30 p.m.

If It Is fried, Then Hide!

Do not even let fried foods see your Bod. They will attack and bring fat back. Have discipline: decide to cut down or not eat fried foods at all.

Don't Bite the White

The *Consumer's Guide* has a great health magazine. One of the rules it promotes is that if it is white, don't bite. This refers to sugars and bleached or white flour breads. Make the decision to limit the whites for a tighter Bod.

Instant Gratification or Fatification?

Instant Fatification vs. long term gratification: Just as people make impulse decisions to purchase an item, people also make impulse decisions when deciding on Fugly foods. You always have several options when deciding whether to eat the candy bar. When this occurs and you think you are about to make an FU decision, **step back and think about the Fatifications**. How will it make you feel in the long term? Is it worth it? Talk yourself out of making that bad FU decision—run, walk, do anything. Call a friend, visit a park, play a game, go shopping. Generate choices instead of fat on your Bod!

Think of cause and effect, action and reaction. You have skipped desserts, and so your reward may be slipping into the pants you could not wear before. You will begin to find that it feels good to make decisions to get to your BB goal, and it feels bad when you make decisions that cause you to wear Fat Ugly.

What Are Your Fat Five?

There is an ad that makes it an honor to be in someone's "Fab Five" phone speed dials. **With Fat Warriors, try planning for five FU decisions per month.** There is no cutting out any foods. You can eat a McDonald's cheeseburger and fries, ice cream, a Twinkie, or anything else five times a month as planned FU decisions. In essence, you have five treats per month or about one per week. This way you give up nothing, but you control the FU decisions. Later you may cut down your FU decisions to three. It may, however, have the danger of the martini rule--one is not enough and two is too many. What are your Fat Five decisions?

Change to making BB decisions and the pain of turning down the ice cream, cake, pastries and SuperSizeMyButt portions eventually goes away. Keep turning down the sweet treats, and simultaneously you will begin turning down the pain of missing them. This key concept is that the pain goes away as the lifestyle change begins.

Eye on the Decisions Ball to Hit Your Right Size

In baseball and softball, coaches teach players that the art of hitting begins with keeping your eye on the ball. You just can't be a good hitter without keeping your eye on the ball.

To hit your personal Right Size, you must have your eye on the ball. That ball is **decisions!** It is not food, scales or calorie counting. Assuming you know the difference between an apple and a brownie, your eye must focus on the decision to go with the apple. If your eye focuses on scales and calorie counting, you will be thinking about the brownie and it will dominate your thoughts and find your mouth. You will see the brownie instead of the apple. You get the picture.

When you do not have your eye on the decisions ball, you will not hit your Right Size. You will be FatStyling forever. To win your war, your thoughts must be on the decision to have the apple over the brownie, the 6-inch lean sub over the 12-inch five-meat sub, or a satisfying portion over a stuffed full portion.

Remember: eye on the decisions ball, not scales or calories. War Face on. You know what is good and bad!

Rule of Positive Decisions: When I make a positive decision, I feel positive and look good. The more positive decisions I make, the better I feel and look.

Rule of Negative Decisions: When I make a negative decision, I feel bad and negative thoughts dominate. The more negative decisions I make, the worse I feel in a downward emotional spiral.

Stand Up to Strawberry Shortcake

Maybe you are just a coward and afraid to stand up to strawberry shortcake. Eating the strawberry fatcake is easy. **If you think about it that way, you will find making BB decisions challenging, but worth the positive outcomes.** Making the decision to say no to ice cream is much easier when you tack on a loss in love life, heart attack, stroke, or diabetes. Take on the battle. Show your War Face and growl. You will **scare the ice cream back into the cone.**

You may think that you will die when you first start making BB decisions, but not eating ice cream for a month won't kill you. Making FU decisions may be easy with instant taste gratification, but afterwards long-term depression sets in. Remember, you are at war with fat. The fact is that these fat decisions also actually kill people and are trying to kill you.

Illuminate, Not Eliminate, All Fuglies

Illuminate your life with understanding and controlling Fuglies, but don't think you must completely eliminate them. Not making any FU decisions is not sustainable or realistic behavior toward living a full life. Your goal should never be to eliminate all Fuglies, but rather to gain total control for a positive balance by constantly improving until you make BB decisions your dominant lifestyle. It is just reversing what made you Fat Ugly. **Your goal is to improve constantly one BB decision at a time, one day at a time, all the time.**

By decreasing your Fuglies and increasing your BB Average, you will move slowly but naturally from Fat Ugly toward Beautiful Bod. So make the decision to cut out the junk and go for lean alternatives instead. By keeping track of your Fatting Average and BB Average, you will be able to see progress in days won, weeks won, and months won. You will be heading toward sustainable behavior that can be permanent. Reaching your personal Right Size is something you can and must and do for health and happiness.

We expect you are occasionally going to make decisions to indulge in Fuglies. These indulgences will be in YOUR TOTAL CONTROL AND A PART OF YOUR PLAN. Remember, it is in your control not to blow your Best Bod on a bulk calorie fat meal or dessert. Just add fitness and exercise to your lifestyle, read labels, go for lower-fat recipes, eat healthy snacks, and resist extra helpings.

Fat Warriors do not ask you to give up anything except a dominating unhealthy lifestyle of Fat Ugly foods and inactivity.

Relentless on Your BBs

Maybe you can't make all of the BB decisions covered in this book, but you can make some of them! Then you will have momentum to make more, and that will reinforce positive behavior. **Keep your eye on your goal of LGFG and go to that mirror.** It takes one decision at a time, one day at a time, to reach your personal Right Size.

<u>**One Rules**</u>**: One good decision, one less sweet treat, one BB meal, one day at a time, to a better life.**

CHAPTER 11

YOUR HOT BOD MANTRA WORKS SKINNIES ALL DAY

I will become my best personal Right Size. I can, must, and will win my BB.

You Must Mantra

Motivation supplied by others will not work. You must be obsessed to do it. Have a positive attitude and say, "I can and will do this, and nothing can stop me!" **Think of what you want to gain and that will become your Fat Warrior mantra.**

Envision your Hot Bod and say your mantra often. Say it, play it, live it, and take your BB back!

SEND IN YOUR MANTRAS TO
WWW.LIFESTYLEWEIGHTEXPERTS.COM!

There Is No Trying, Only Doing or Not Doing

Do not say to yourself you are going to try to do it or you will fail. You must know you can do it, and that starts with your mantra now! It has been said there is only doing or not doing. Right now, in this moment, what you decide to do or not do will come true. It will not always go perfectly, you will have successes but also some failures and setbacks. You will embrace and build on successes, and acknowledge and learn from the setbacks.

The adventure will make you stronger. You will know that if you never give up you cannot lose, and if you keep fighting you will eventually win. It is a process of life, and that is why our turtle beats the hare. **You simply decide you must and will win. You must mantra!**

CHAPTER 12

HOW BODY, MIND AND SPIRIT BUILD LIFESTYLE OF THIN

Your Body, Mind, and Spirit (BMS) Must Be in Concert

There must be harmony between your Body, Mind, and Spirit (BMS), and you are the conductor who must keep them in tune. A diet or plan cannot conduct your BMS in harmony, so the plans and diets will fail in the search for the BMS Holy Grail of permanent weight loss. Any part of the BMS trinity can overpower the other two parts, derail the quest for your personal Right Size, and stop you from reaching your dreams. The BMS trinity is believed to be so powerful that it cannot be denied and will always make you confident and victorious. **When the Body, Mind, and Spirit are working together, your victory of a permanent Beautiful Bod is assured!**

BMS, Working Together

For example, you decide you want to lose weight and diet. Your Spirit dictates to your Mind and Body that you deprive and cut down on food to lose weight. Eventually, deprivation causes hunger pains, which cause the Mind and Body to override the Spirit's decision to cut down on food, and diet failure occurs. At some point, you are likely to eat so much to satisfy the hunger pains that you gain rebound pounds plus failure depression. The Body, Mind, and Spirit of a dieter not being in sync is one reason that diets so often fail, and the reason why diet plans are removing the word "diet" from their advertising.

The Body, Mind, and Spirit must be in concert to gain your BB by eating nutritious food without starving the Body. You will not experience rebound pounds or the hunger of deprivation if you follow the Fat Warriors program. You will simply be Looking Good, Feeling Good, and feel that you are gaining everything you desire and deserve. Your Body, Mind, and Spirit are anxiously anticipating your future Hot Bod lifestyle.

Your Spirit

You are fighting mad and nothing will stop your victory of taking your BB back. You are just not going to take it anymore. That comes from the journey from your brain to your heart. Is that Mind or Spirit? People say this comes from the heart and can be so strong as to influence the brain into positive action and the Bod follows the direction. Your will and what we think of as a higher purpose must be the Spirit. **You have a strong Spirit, and if you use it, it can win many wonderful things for you.** Pray, chant, think, go for a higher purpose, and live your positive Self-Talk into your beliefs. Whether you think you can or can't, you are probably right. We know you can!

You've Got Spirit, Yes You Do!

Your can-do Spirit responds with more mind muscle and motivation by self-competition when FU and BB decisions are being measured and recorded. The fact is that when you're scoring your BBs and FUs, this powers the Body and Mind to go to great lengths to meet goals. It is difficult to win without scoring. This is the secret in business and why goal setting and measuring progress works. It is said in business that what gets measured and recorded gets done. If there is no record, there is less fanfare and applause. If there are no measurements, productivity is not likely to be achieved and underachievement occurs.

59

In almost anything, the Spirit of competition spurs better performance and results. Make participation in Fat Warriors a fun game by making it a competition with points scored for goals met. Get groups together for even more fun competing against one another or as teams. Use your BMS trinity to get your game on!

If Your Diet Is Not Sustainable, That Will Mean Eat the Table

Your Bod will demand to eat, so starving it or dieting is likely not sustainable behavior. When you deprive your Bod, it overrides the Mind and Spirit.

The Bod will keep sending messages to the brain to eat and eat a lot in case you starve it again. It stores up Fat Ugly protection in case of another starving period. So when you start to lose weight, you are setting your Bod up for rebound pounds and a minefield of depression, tears, and sadness. So the Bod can override the Mind and Spirit? Think about it.

Visualize, Breathe, See, Hear, Feel

The entire process is owned and run by you, your Body, Mind, and Spirit. **By focusing on your BMS instead of pills and calorie counting, your chances for successfully attaining a healthy lifestyle are much higher.**

CHAPTER 13

PYRAMIDS OF LIFESTYLE CHANGE

Up Yours! Taking Baby Steps Up Your Lifestyle Pyramid

Begin with baby steps by gradually making more BBs. You will follow the pyramid of the Hot Bod to the level that is right for you. You don't need to get there quickly, just take baby steps that make sense to you. Trust us! **You will naturally progress to better health if you follow the pyramid as high as you wish to go.**

Find what works for you, and you will always be improving one baby step at a time. Example: Start taking baby steps up the pyramid by choosing less processed food. You do this by cutting back on canned and packaged food and eating more fresh meats, veggies, and fruits instead. You are consciously making decisions to eat more foods found around the perimeter of the grocery store, where the healthier foods are found, rather than in the middle of the store, where the FU foods are located. Recording the FU and BB decisions in your grocery cart will help you bring home Bod Hot foods to eat and not wear.

Now is the time to start taking baby steps up the pyramid. As you ascend one level at a time, you will retrain your Body, Mind, and Spirit to be in concert within 30-90 days. You will then have gained a fun lifestyle change that you will love.

Start Pyramiding one level at a time until you get to the level that is best for you!

CHAPTER 14

EAT NAKED
MAKING LOVE TO YOUR
FOOD

FatCrap

FatCrap is defined as undesired chemicals and additives placed into foods. **FatCrap is an ugly name for ugly chemicals and additives.**

Chemicals and additives may make fruits, vegetables, cattle, poultry and pigs fatter and plumper faster for slaughter. Might you be becoming fatter and plumper faster because of these same additives? These additives are used to grow, plump up, fat up, preserve, and do things to foods that are not natural. They may be called things like hormones, steroids, preservatives and fertilizer. I just call ugly chemicals FatCrap that may be SuperSizing you. These FatCrap additives may be labeled with names you cannot pronounce or define their purpose.

You may be putting FatCrap undesirables into your Body without even knowing their harm. Nature did not intend or desire FatCrap for your healthy Bod.

Avoid FatCrap and Still Enjoy the Taste

Don't ruin a salad by putting FatCrap dressings to excess on it. Fat-loaded salad dressing will undress all the good the salad might bring. Examples include any dressing with cheese in the name. Eating salads or meats that are bathed in saucy chemicals is just fattening. I did not feel that way until I became the Fat Warrior and learned from the Food Strippers and Naked Eaters to avoid many chemicals in dressings

63

and sauces for the goal of Right Sizing. **The fact is that after a while you will figure out a way to eat all things with less chemicals and still enjoy the taste.** You just will not have to deal with the after-fat.

Free Range Animals Taste Better!

You would definitely want to eat free-range beef after visiting a stench-filled feedlot. It is gut wrenching to visit a cattle feedlot where the cattle are raised in pens and fed at a trough. The food is akin to pig slop, and instead of grazing on grass they eat from the trough. It is filled with FatCrap containing chemicals, steroids, and antibiotics with grains mixed in. It would shock you to observe how the penned up, trough fed, chemically grown cattle are lazy, seem depressed and have no energy.

In 2005, famous newsman Bill Kurtis founded a large operation for free-range cattle. It is not free cattle, but I will pay for the extra value of more natural meat. Consider buying meat from free range cattle, pigs, and buffalo. Consider the health benefits, both mental and physical. If you observe cattle in a feedlot as opposed to free range, you may become a free ranger too. There is a song that says, "Home, home on the range, where the deer and the antelope play..." There is no doubt in the Fat Warrior's mind that animals that are allowed to move, forage and graze are leaner, healthier and happier than their FatCrap-fed counterparts.

Eat Raw?

Ponder this: Nature did not intend for us to eat chemicals and additives. Wild animals eat raw meat and other foods and are not fat unless man interferes. People love sushi, but of course humans would become ill by eating some foods raw, such as chicken, etc. **Sticking as close to nature as possible with**

natural foods minus the chemicals will benefit the Body, Mind, and Spirit and result in a leaner Bod.

It is known that cooking takes nutrients out of foods, but it also kills bacteria and other things that can be harmful. The Fat Warrior likes to cook things in a Crock-Pot, thereby keeping the natural juices in. I sometimes wonder what eating would be like without the stove, microwave and fast foods. Something to stew over in my Crock-Pot.

Naked Eating

Eating Naked means eating foods that are "naked" of FatCrap unhealthy chemicals. It is about eating more fresh fruits, vegetables, and whole grains, and removing toxic chemicals from your Bod. Eating Naked by removing or cutting back on processed foods in your diet is great for your Body, Mind, and Spirit. Many experts agree that Eating Naked will expose your Bod to healthier foods, and as a result you will become healthier and smaller.

Which Type of Naked Eating Is Right for You?

There are three levels of Eating Naked and they all deal with getting bare and exposing your Bod.

The first level is exposing and stripping yourself of your old thoughts and Fabits that have contributed to your current Fat Ugly lifestyle.

The second level is beginning to strip away the chemicals and additives in the foods you eat by eating more fresh fruits, vegetables, and whole grains. This is the most important principle of Eating Naked. It means counting chemicals that may be more harmful than calories. Try beginning to strip processed foods from your diet and trade them for fresh foods. We call this level "semi-nude," as Fat Warriors in this category may not be comfortable going completely naked. These Naked Eaters are aware of what is going into their Bods and try to make a gradual shift to a healthier diet.

The third level may be the most fun, is literally Eating Naked. Naked Eaters in this category have completely removed chemical-laden foods from their diets and gone organic.

Eating Naked and FantaSizing

Eating Naked and FantaSizing while doing it can be pleasurable and fun with positive rewards. Eating Naked while FantaSizing may carry a mature rating and should only be done by consenting adults. It can be done in the kitchen, dining room, and even the bedroom. The foreplay starts in your mind and is executed at the grocery store or market!

I always FantaSize while Eating Naked. My fantasies are made up of positive visions of what I want my Bod and lifestyle to be. I have FantaSized to a 34 inch waist from a 38. I have FantaSized away my fat stomach, man boobs, and 15 pounds by Eating Naked and FantaSizing. Eating Naked decisions grew on me and my Fat Ugly started wilting.

Eating Naked is easy to get used to and will grow on you as you accomplish the goals of an energetic lifestyle of LGFG.

Naked Eaters' Conversations

Naked Eaters all have one thing in common. They have upbeat attitudes and brag about their activities and lifestyle. Instead of talking about diets and misery, Naked Eaters talk about how much they eat and how happy they are. For example: Naked Eater woman says, "I can wear my high school jeans." Her friend retorts, "I can wear my high school jeans also, but they fit a little loose." The third friend says, "I can wear the pair of jeans that I got when I was two, but they are a little short." Then they all laugh as Right-Sizers have their fun.

Naked Eater man says, "My stomach looks as flat as an aircraft carrier." His dad replies, "I have lost my man boobs." The man's brother says, "I have so much energy, yesterday I jumped over my car and today I will jump over my house."

Right-Sizers have great senses of humor and talk upbeat about life. **Sure, they have problems, but Right-Sizers are not obsessed with talking dieting or thinking about depriving themselves of everything but pity. They laugh at fat people looking at the before and after pictures to select their next fat failure diet plan.** Diets just cannot muscle up to the fun and success of Eating Naked and FantaSizing.

Jamaica Naked Phenomenon

The most fascinating, pleasant thing happened while staying in Jamaica at an all-inclusive resort. Everybody ate breakfast, lunch and dinner, plus snacks. Most of us were having drinks at lunch and drinks under the hot sun while on the beach. Nighttime was feast and party time. At the end of the vacation, many people could not believe they had not gained a lot of weight. I have observed this phenomenon after years of traveling to Jamaica and have come to a remarkable conclusion.

I finally figured out the Jamaica phenomenon. We were all Eating Naked without realizing it. The food was all grown fresh, the meat came from grass-fed animals in Jamaica, and the fish were fresh from the ocean. This was my first great experience of eating almost free of FatCrap and not gaining weight. It was certifiably wonderful to experience great food without FatCrap and weight gain.

If you believe as I do, then as they say on the beaches of Jamaica, go "au naturel." Eat natural foods as much as possible. I have never seen a field of Ding Dongs or Twinkies growing on a farm. That means they are processed foods. **Try to eat more of the foods that Mother Nature grew for you free of chemicals and fewer processed foods. If it is** natural, you will know it when you see it, so give it a try!

Island Eating

I also observed the Jamaica phenomenon on Maui. By eating more fruits, veggies, and fish you are Eating Naked and looking lean because of less junk food. Get the junk out of your trunk and island eat. Island eating is like eating the foods on the perimeter of your supermarket. Think of the perimeter foods at the grocery store as the beach. Select foods from the beach and they will help you get your Beach Bod back! Imagine the reggae music and envision your Hot Bod as you score BBs into your cart!

Bourbon Street Poundage

I found the opposite when I spent a week in New Orleans. I came back with bloated water weight and extra fat poundage. Unlike Jamaica, in New Orleans my Bod paid dearly for the vacation. I was definitely not Eating Naked in The Big Easy!

Seduce Your Food!

Hand in hand with Eating Naked, Fat Warriors make love to their food. By engaging in foreplay with your food, it will last longer, so you will eat less. Let the tongue taste and have an affair with the meal. French kiss your food as you experience tingles of good taste on your tongue. Tease your food as you fork it up. Take time and look at the presentation of colors, smell it, and the five senses will take over. Let the flavors burst in your mouth, take your time before swallowing.

Fall in love with your food. This romantic experience allows you to enjoy food more, but because of the seduction time you will eat less. Take time to savor the flavor!

> *Make love to your food and seduce it slowly with foreplay. If you have fun with your food and take time to love it, then you will eat more slowly. Slowly savor it, chew it, taste it.*

Chemical Free for Me?

The Lifestyle Weight Experts Team does not suggest that you must go entirely chemical free, but we believe that you should begin making more fresh eating part of your lifestyle. Baby steps for your Body, Mind, and Spirit!

Eating fresh foods that are grown locally and products from grass-fed animals will eliminate many bad chemicals. Going chemical free may help you obtain your best nourishment, your best mood, best health, and provide you with your personal best Beautiful Bod to show off.

Find your starting point. Dip your toes in the Naked, fresh waters, try a few things, and see if you want to begin swimming in chemical-free health!

CHAPTER 15

ORGANIC SKINNY BABY STEPS

Decisions are grown in the mind, provided by the harvest of thought seeds, and are 100 percent organic. No fertilizers, you are directly responsible for your Fat Ugly or BB decisions.

Eat Fresh

The easy way to become a Naked Eater is to consume more organic foods and fewer processed foods. Since writing books and developing the Fat Warriors Nation, the Fat Warrior has been cutting down on processed food and eating more organic fresh foods instead.

I am not an organic nutcase, but an organic suitcase. Organic decisions seem to suit me better the more I make them. I fell in love with eating more fresh food. You may find as I have that the investment in eating fresh and more organic pays off in gaining looks, health, wealth, and self-esteem.

> *The items found in the middle of the grocery store will fill your cart full of the Fat Ugliest processed foods. These middle-of-the-store foods have an infinite shelf life and will ride on your butt forever.*

Eat Like You Flirt - Fresh

It is amazing that when we start grazing on fresh vegetables, fruits, nuts, and other nutritious snacks we start looking Bod Hot great and feeling super.

Try fresh flirting. Start with small things like eating more fresh fruits and veggies, and after about 30 days you will actually start preferring greens to cans. Can the cans because it works! I did not believe it at first, but I did it and now there are far fewer cans and processed foods that will outlast dirt in my house.

Train the brain to prefer fresh and you will feel livelier, smile bigger and jump over tall buildings.

What Is Your IQ?

Replace calorie counting with your Ingredient Quota (IQ). Your Ingredient Quota is not based on anything related to your brain IQ. Or is it?

What is your harmful IQ of how many and what chemicals you will allow to be added per food or package? Determine your IQ by counting the number of additives before counting the package out.

Organic Does Not Mean Organic, Or Does It?

You read the label and it says it's organic, but does that mean it really is organic? Unravel the mystery clues by knowing the three key organic labels:

Label 1: "100% Organic"

- This means an ingredient list must be displayed as well as the organic certifier. You should not see any chemicals or additives, etc., as they are not allowed in 100% organic products. Example: Grapes in a package labeled "100% Organic" will list the ingredient as ... grapes. Yep, just grapes.

Label 2: "USDA Organic"

- For this level, the contents must only match up to 95% organic ingredients. That leaves 5% that can be additives, chemicals, synthetics, etc. The label must contain the organic certifier's name and list the non-organic components.

Label 3: "Made with Organic"

- If you read the label as "Made with Organic," it must contain 70% organic ingredients and the name of the certifier. I am not comfortable with this label because I have no idea if 70% is good or bad, but it may be better than no rating.

If you look at it as a health investment, organic is the better investment for your Body, Mind, and Spirit.

Does Organic Eating Cost More?

It may at first blush, but I think I can show you why organic eating may be cheaper! The organic investment may pay off big time in less fat, depression, and tiredness in exchange for Looking Good, Feeling

Good. How much would you pay for a pill that made you look good and feel good?

There are many larger issues as well. Diminished health costs alone may pay for eating organic. Add the costs of things like sickness, missed work, diabetes, and anti-depressives. Factor in the cost of buying clothes for hoggers, and organic food becomes a bargain! Look at the difference in the size of fruits that are enhanced by chemical growing as compared to certified organic. **That big, fat, plump fruit may be fattening you up and those big jeans cost a lot. You will likely start eating smaller portions when you eat organic, partly because organic food is so nutritious and will satisfy your needs with less.**

We can have spirited debates about whether eating organic may be cheaper in the long run of life.

Health Nuts?

You may think eating organic is only for health nuts. I did, too. Although organics eat nuts in the raw, they are not nuts. The logic of adding chemicals to fruits, vegetables, and meats is easy to understand. Chemicals act as preservatives, pickling the food to last longer than Mother Nature would naturally allow. **If your foods last longer than my run-on sentences, they contain chemical preservatives. Don't be pickled by them.**

CHAPTER 16

RABBIT AND TURTLE
WEIGHT RACE

Think Slow
You have learned that the only way to lose weight permanently is to take a slow and steady approach to achieving lifestyle changes. **The slower fat comes off, the longer it stays off. If you lose it too quickly, it will return quickly, which usually brings extra rebound pounds.** So don't be discouraged at steady, successful progress in your battle to Right Size; stay focused on making positive lifestyle decisions that will help you achieve your goal of Right Sizing for life!

Baby Steps First
Start with baby steps, don't go for 100 pounds right away. Just begin with BB decisions that result in permanent lifestyle changes, which in turn cause slow weight loss, one pound at a time, that you will keep off forever. Don't think of it as losing one pound, but instead gaining Looking Good and Feeling Fantastic. Visualize looking hot as your belt reduces notches. Lose Fabits, not weight. Gain the positive things you desire for you!

So begin with easy BBs. Make positive decisions on foods which will possibly become your first lifestyle changes. Get moving, forward march!

Starting Sustainable Change
Decisions to make behavioral changes, whether portion size, selection of food or exercise, must be sustainable to be maintainable. Self-reliant turtle

speed works best. Rabbit speed is non-sustainable behavior; you can't run at full speed for the long run.

As a Fat Warrior you are committing to a new approach to changing your lifestyle. Lifestyle changes don't happen overnight for permanent sustainability. We are here to help, with ideas and tools that provide guidance for sustainable behavior to a new Best Bod lifestyle.

Think about gaining a winning lifestyle for the long term, and your progress over time will be permanent.

Recommit, Don't Quit!

Keep score and have fun. Just start with a base hit as one good BB decision replaces a bad FU decision. Your base hits will become grand slam homers of sustainable lifestyle changes over time.

Keeping score and averaging is the most important tool to get you to your Right Size. Keep scoring BBs and FUs until your BB Average is consistently above 750. This may take several months. Be patient, don't quit. The objective is permanent weight loss, not quick and easy weight loss, which sets you up for fat to return. Turtle speed wins!

CHAPTER 17

POWER YOUR NOW MOMENT NOW

The only moment and decisions that you control are in the now. What you are doing in the now, right now, is determining your future Bod size and lifestyle.

Now Is the Pow

The decisions you make now foretell your Bod of tomorrow. The now moment is all you control. If you deal with your decisions right now, you can overpower your Fat Ugly and be on your way to a slimmer, happier and healthier tomorrow.

If you don't start changing now, you will carry forth the same problem for your entire future, feeling Fat Ugly plus getting older. It is much more fun to age gracefully with a smile and Looking Good, Feeling Good in your Beautiful Bod.

Start focusing on the now; now for pow!

Pleasures of the Now vs. LGFG Future

Many people put their fat pleasures on the front burner. The back burner gets the discipline to say No. For these people, their future Bod is not even on the stove. Do you want the pleasure of now, or the consequences of the future? Do you want to pay for the temporary fat pleasure of minutes now instead of the LGFG permanence of the future? Instead of feeling you need that candy bar treat now, get up and run or walk, but move out now! Invest in your future now and you will feel better!

NOW Is the Rest of Your Lifestyle!

Tomorrows are made in the now moment, so start now for your future BB lifestyle. Yesterday's gone, tomorrow is not today, now will play forever in your life. You have won your first victory by buying and starting this book. So ride the now, now. (That is enough now for right now.)

CHAPTER 18

BE AWARE,
DON'T WEAR FAT CLOTHES
FOREVER

Fat Warriors Awareness Rule: If you are not aware of your FU decisions, then you will wear them and have to SuperSize your clothes.

Eat and Wear

Every time you make a Fat Ugly decision, you will have a few minutes of temporary taste pleasure, followed by hours of wishing you had not made that choice. You will have days of low self-esteem as you wear your fat to work and waddle around your community. You have heard of wash and wear; this is eat and wear. Think of the ratio of the fat pleasure compared to the pain ratio. There is no comparison. You are trading minutes of pleasure for days, weeks, or years of painful depression. Think of years of fat tears. Years or 15 minutes, you decide.

Grasp the truth until it is engrained into your brain about this bad ratio of pleasure taste to fatness pain. The truth will power your thoughts and become your belief that you can win your personal Right Size. You can make the right decisions and keep making more of them until they become habit. That is the truth, but you must believe and not be a Doubting Thomas.

> **Rule of Taste**: If it tastes good, then I must treat myself to one. In a matter of minutes the good taste is gone and the bad feelings linger, as does the fat, forever. You wear what you eat. The fact is that fat foods taste good temporarily, but make you feel bad forever.

Treats Lead to Defeats

You look at that ice cream cone, currently one of your favorite Fat Ugly delights. If you are Fat Ugly, then you have programmed your brain into wanting it and getting it. What a wonderful pleasure for ten minutes, and then there is a wave of disappointment in yourself as you understand you are wearing those Fugly pleasures for life.

Rewarding yourself with something to make you fat doesn't make sense and is counter-productive for your visualized goal of attaining your personal Right Size. Fat treats should be something you have once in a while and in small portions.

Do not associate ice cream, whipped cream, candy bars, cake or pizza with rewards. Their only trophy is a fat stomach instead of flat stomach.

If your treats are based on fat food pleasures like brownies and chocolate bars, then you are training your mind to associate treats and rewards with something that will kill your self-esteem, participation in life, and your life.

It's Not Always As It Appears

It is a myth that people in big houses with shiny new things are always happy. It may be a false belief, as they may be deep in mortgage debt, carry a heavy payment load, or high credit card debt. Maybe they work long days and weekends to make the big house happen and don't have time to enjoy life. Possessions may have become their life and are causing them misery.

You imagine the ice cream will be so wonderful and very enjoyable, but it is growing that Fat Ugly mortgage payment and debt of your butt and health. You possess all the good tasting things, but they are killing your possibility of a healthy life when you wear them. **The Happy Meal may look happy, but may provide a sad life.**

Items in Your Pantry You Will Wear

Your pantry features what your mouth will pant for when you open it. Notice that the pantry shelves reflect your grocery store decisions. You carry the items from the store, put them in the pantry, and they are ready to wear. Your pantry can also be loaded with nutritional Beautiful Bod decisions leading to looking good in clothes. What's in your pantry?

You Wear What You Eat

Live more aware of what you are doing now and the great things you want your Beautiful Bod to be. Be aware of what you eat or don't eat, whether you exercise or not. Being aware of these decisions, actions and their consequences is the only way you can optimize your ability to control them. **Awareness leads to your ability to control your decisions and that is mandatory for your success.**

Concentrate on awareness or you may miss many super opportunities to do good things for you. Years ago I was a deer hunter. You quickly learn that you must focus or you will not even see the deer. By concentrating and being aware, a hunter may suddenly see a deer or many deer blending into the foliage. I learned that if I saw one deer, more were usually there that would become visible.

Be aware of your thoughts, feelings, and beliefs while you eat. Make them positive and filled with dreams of wonderful things happening to your Beautiful Bod. If you are aware of your intentions, then you probably won't pull onto the SuperSizeMyButt highway.

CHAPTER 19

SCORE YOUR GROCERY CART.
TODAY SEE YOUR BOD OF TOMORROWS.

Does your grocery cart scream, "I belong to a fat person," or "I belong to a Hot Bod"?

Home Houses Grocery Cart Decisions

What is in your grocery cart goes into your house, then your mouth, and then you wear it. **The grocery cart tells the story of whether you live to eat or eat to live.** What you put in the cart dictates where you go to buy your clothes, what you look like, feel like, and your health.

You have stocked your home with what you look like. If you hide foods to fool anybody, you will only be fooling the fool and hurting yourself. So get it out in the open for you and everyone to see your selections. You will be proud to display good food that will help you look good.

Never Fill Grocery Carts with Groceries!

Check in for life or check out of life at the grocery store check stand. The items going down the conveyor belt to the cashier are not groceries! Yes, they look like groceries, you are charged for them as groceries, and people call them groceries, but they are not groceries. **Grocery carts are filled with *decisions.***

ScoreBook Your Grocery Cart Decisions
Before you go grocery shopping, your action plan might start by making a list and sticking with it. For a better score keep score, record, and compare your grocery cart Fuglies and BBs week to week for six months. You win the battle of the grocery cart and your belt-buckling victory is in sight!

Grocery Stores Are Stocked Full of BBs and Fuglies
Grocery shopping presents many decisions opportunities when selecting foods to cart home. If you decide to buy ice cream, whipped cream, sugar cereals, potato chips, and candy disguised as food, they are all your decisions to make you Fat Ugly.

Put FU decisions in your grocery cart to cart home for growing your gigantic figure. Put BB decisions in the cart to dance home and embrace your Looking Good figure of tomorrow. Which do you choose? Score yourself one BB for the decision not to select predominantly FU foods, as well as for the decision to purchase BB foods.

Packaged Food May Mean Packaged Fatness
Packages do not grow on trees, and farmers are not harvesting fields of boxes and packages. **If food comes in a box or package, there is a good chance it is processed food, which may make your packaging fatter.** Be aware. Fresh foods make you fresher. If Mother Nature grew them, then she meant

you to look good wearing them. Cupcakes do not grow in fields, so put the packaged fat stuff back now.

Grocery Carts Filled with Fabits and Grabits

Think first, before you grab. If you purchase BBs instead of Fuglies, you are stocking your home with healthy food that will make you and your loved ones look and feel great. In the long run, they will appreciate you for it. You will also save money by not purchasing expensive junk food that causes you to eat more.

Remember the potato chip that claimed the fame of you can't eat just one?

Cart Peeping Can Be Fun *and* Legal

People are checking out your big-out grocery selections or your healthy foods. A good nutritionist could probably look at a grocery cart and guess the Bod style of the owner. Look at grocery carts and then look at their owners.   Are they TrimStylers or FatStylers?

Cart peeping can be fun and a learning experience. Play the game, peek at the cart, and guess the weight of the cart pusher. The closest wins an apple.

Your Grocery Cart Is the Predictor of Your Future Looks and Feelings

Your grocery cart outweighs your scale with impact on your Right Size. **Look at your grocery cart instead of your scale**. Grocery cart decisions eat scales for breakfast and munch on calorie counters. Do you fill your cart with Fuglies or BBs? Your scale's Bod impact score is zero, but your grocery cart scores dramatic Bod effects.

What is on the checkout conveyor belt is conveying your future Beautiful Bod, or belting out your waistline.

What you see in the grocery cart is the future story of your FU or BB Bod.

CHAPTER 20

EXCUSES AND DOUBTS
BUILD PERMANENT FAT UGLY

Fat Warriors Affirmation
_Fat Warriors means NO WHINING. WHINING IS
NOT TAUGHT IN THIS BOOK. Excuses are not
allowed in Fat Warrior Boot Camp. Can't do is
out. Feeling sorry is allowed only when talking
to your priest, mother or bartender. There is
no entitlement mentality in Fat Warriors.
Whining hides when there is a War Face and
growl present._

FU Example of Victim Mentality

"I believe that my pig-out rituals provide me with
such pleasure that I can't win my war on fat. I am a fat
victim of my parents, my government, McDonald's, ice
cream, my own willpower, and so I have resigned to
stay fat. I can prove it. I have lost weight but always
gained it back. My belief is that I can't win, and my
reaction is to give up and give in. I will make FU
decisions because I am loaded with excuses and am
weak. So pass the pie and add a dose of ice cream
topped with whipped cream. No, I said pass the pie,
not a piece of pie, the _pie_."

Blame Game and Excuses

Blame your fatness on the spoon, genetics, the President, or that you're too busy to eat healthy. Blame gives you wonderful excuses for eating like a pig for temporary enjoyment and permanent miserable esteem. If you tell the Fat Warrior you are feeling fine being fat, then eat a cookie and go see a psychiatrist.

Fat Warriors discard excuses and leave them for negative underachievers for comfort food of the mind. Excuses and alibis are luxuries of fat people and people who want to feel good about feeling bad and failing. How about some Excuse Mousse or Alibi Pie?

> *I can't, this is just the way I am--fat. I have no willpower and so I am happy being fat. It's not my fault.*

Excuses for Not Trying or Failing

We spend all of our mental muscle championing our excuses and supporting our victim mentality. We limit other possibilities because it is better to be right than happy. I've never seen a fat person with excuses lose weight permanently. I've never seen a thin person who had any excuses. Think about it and you may want to dump your Fat Ugly by dumping your excuses.

There are thousands of excuses and they are the best thing for giving you reasons to accept failure instead of trying. **Excuses are wonderful feel-good reasons for giving up and not succeeding.** You must exchange excuses for perseverance, seasoned with a refusal to give up if you want to win your personal Right Size.

Don't Tell the Fat Warrior It Is Too Hard to Give Up Your Fat Ugly Lifestyle

You just may be a sissy when you make the excuse that making BB decisions is too hard. Think of all the traumas that you go through being Fat Ugly. Now *that's* hard! If you think about it that way, you will FIGHT TO POWER MORE BB DECISIONS. The more you make, the better you will feel about yourself.

Puke Out Your Favorite Excuses

Put your excuses down on paper. List them, puke them out, and get them out of your thinking system. Define your Top 10 excuses and either accept them and your fate, or kick them out of your mind and off your fat behind. **Put on your War Face, stare your excuses down, and then send them to our website at www.lifestyleweightexperts.com. You can join us in making a list of the best Fataholic Excuses!**

Your Imaginary Wheelbarrow

Your imaginary wheelbarrow is currently filled with excuses that will prevent you from winning your BB. So dump your imaginary wheelbarrow of excuses out and into the trash, and instead fill it with can-do's, Right-Sizing decisions, health visions, Beautiful Bod dreams, etc. When it is emptied of negative thoughts and excuses and refilled with positive beliefs, you are in a position to succeed!

You Must Do More Than Show Up

If you do not want to play, then don't come to the playground. If you want to make excuses and your mode is negative, then don't! Don't do the deal, don't interview, don't go to the party. Don't become a Fat Warrior unless you want to, otherwise stay on the couch along with your Fat Ugly excuses and watch.

CHAPTER 21

SELF-ESTEEM UP:
EAT TO LIVE – FOR SEX,
HEALTH, AND WEALTH

Make it your goal to live life, not eat it!

If You Eat to Live, Most of Your Life and Time Will Be Directed at Having Fun and Owning Your Desires

We base this theory on the fact that you spend a total of about one hour a day actually engaging the mouth in eating. Now, oinkers may spend more time than that, but the dilemma exists. **This means you counteract one hour of fun eating tasty pleasures by 23 hours of feeling embarrassed, bloated, ugly, fat, sluggish, tired, and weak.** You do the math, and you may want to fight back. Be a Fat Warrior and enjoy the 23 hours instead of one hour oinking.

Treat or Retreat?

Beautiful Bods believe in the paradigm of eating to live lively. They do not believe in gorging themselves with all the tasty morsels that get in their way of happiness. They deliberately select when to treat and when to retreat. They live for the 23 hours of the day when they own Looking Good, Feeling Good. The mirror is their friend, and they make friends more easily with the opposite sex. **Do you need to be a rocket scientist to figure the math of 23 hours vs. 1 hour?**

It is a small price to pay to change your paradigm from living to eat to eating to live. Think about it: enjoying minutes of taste pleasure vs. hours and days of LGFG, getting the girl or guy, getting the job, and getting your smile back.

Weigh That Thought

Do your Fat Ugly decisions currently outweigh your dreams of an LGFG lifestyle? If so, that is why you are now FU. It is not the food you're eating, it is your decisions of living to eat. Only when a paradigm shift occurs and eating to live becomes more important than your desire to gorge yourself will you self-motivate to achieve the goal of your personal Right Size. It will take perseverance but you can, will, and must do it.

Beautiful Bod people have a fun life before, during, and after food! **The astonishing thing is that BBs probably enjoy good food more than hoggers enjoy Fugly foods.** Fuglies can learn to like fruits, vegetables, lean meats, and less fattening foods. Beautiful Bods like them, and so will you if you try. You will find that some BBs eat things with weird names like tofu, but they also eat beef and everything else in right-sized portions. Their dominant thinking is for health and happiness. **Sprinkle moderation on anything and it becomes a little better.**

CHAPTER 22

WHY SCALES PROMOTE FAT THINKING

Scales have the power to get you to step on them, read them, and think of weighing as an important thing to do.

Riddle: What effect does scale weighing have on helping you lose fat? **Answer:** Since you bought a scale, it has caused you to lose nothing except money and time.

We believe that you must get off the scale, as it has never gotten the weight off of you. If scales helped people lose weight, then they would sell like diamonds. How much would you pay for a scale that played a role in winning your Beautiful Bod?

Weighing is just not working--ask the professional yo-yo dieter. Fat Warriors replace the scale with your ScoreCard and mirror. Put the scale in the closet and bring it out once a month. It can be useful for a monthly weight check, which means clearly that you are in it for the long term and permanent change.

Your Goal Is Not Weighed in Pounds, but in Smiles

Have you ever weighed a smile? Even if you add pride and sprinkles of participating activities, the weight of a smile remains the same.

As a Fat Warrior you must program your mind that your goal is not simply weight loss, but gaining your personal Right Size. You must program your mind to go from a Fat Ugly lifestyle of depression and avoidance to a lifestyle of joy and happiness and participating. Your goal is not measured in poundage but in joy. Have a scale measure smiles and we can talk. Leave the scale behind; you are gaining your personal Right Size and a better life.

Fat laughs at scales and calorie counters, so count them out and toss them out.

Scale Distraction

You wake up and go to the scale to see if you have lost weight. You are happy if you lost weight, even though you have been down this road before and gained it back. Now you focus on the scale and weight loss. That is sad, looking down constantly thinking of losing weight.

Instead of looking down at your scale, wake up, look up, and review yesterday's decisions on your ScoreCard and tallies for the week. Plan the positive decisions that you will make today. Approach the day with a can-do, "I am the decision-maker" mindset. **Wake up, put on your makeup, and get ready to go to war for your better life.**

As you go through your day, count the BB decisions that are leading toward a lifestyle change and a healthier, sexier Bod. Count the FU decisions that are keeping you in fat depression. Focus on making decisions that will lead you to your personal Right Size. **Step off the scale and step up decision scoring! Weigh in with BBs rather than a scale.**

Scale Tossing As a Sport and Being a Sport
Toss your scale out as far as you can, you do not want it under your feet to distract you. We call this scale tossing. You may toss it in the trash or toss it to your neighbor, but toss it out! (At least toss it into the closet, and only bring it out once per month.) Keep it out of sight, out of mind.

Instead of standing on a scale every day and looking down, hold your head up and do the scale toss. You will understand why the scale is a diversion that causes you to lose your focus on BB decisions and scoring, and why it may have many negative effects on your ultimate goal of a better life.

Scale tossing can be fun when you toss a perfectly good scale to your neighbor. Then explain the Fat Warriors strategy behind scale tossing. Toss this paragraph around the neighborhood.

If your girth suggests birth, you don't need a scale to see it.

CHAPTER 23

GET OFF THE COUCH
TO GET WEIGHT OFF

With no exercise you get the flabbies instead of muscle and become a walking jiggle. Exercise and become a lean, mean fighting machine.
You will look great and feel great!

Move: A Four-Letter Word

You must exercise and that means move! Clean the house, mow the lawn, walk the stairs, walk anywhere, but MOVE. You must get your exercise going in some fashion, even if it is not a fashionable health club. You can even walk in place watching TV. Commit, time it, and do it.

Moving causes your metabolism to burn fat. Movement outruns depression (most of the time), so get off the couch and MOVE!

Endorphins: The Legal High Untaxed

The best high is not from food or drugs, it is from endorphins. Runners call it a "runner's high" and it is not illegal or taxed. (Don't tell Uncle Sam or he will tax it.) Don't let anybody tell you that it costs too much. You can't get a lid, kilo, bag, or prescription. Gangs don't sell it. Endorphins kick funk's ass.

Most will tell you that it is non-addictive. I have no evidence, but I like my endorphin highs so much that I exercise five days a week and enjoy them. Yes, you can drive while under the influence of an endorphin high. Your right brain creative juices will flow and you will bring forth ideas that will make millions. Okay, I am on an endorphin high as I write this.

Sweat Does Not Stink When It Is Yours

Many people have a false belief about exercise. They think it is good for them, but too hard to do for the benefits. They may not see the benefits from their couch. They see running and sweating. I see an endorphin high, creative juices, positive attitude, and a mood elevator when I am down. I see that I am a better performer, happier person, and look and feel better.

Start Slowly

I made a smart decision that I needed some form of exercise to become a part of my life. I was in the shape of about 215 pounds, and in the fattest, worst shape of my life. I looked fat, felt fat, and was fat-out depressed. I decided to do something and started running again. I had not run in four years.

I selected running because it always put me in a positive mood and gave me a great outlook and better problem-solving abilities. Running is easy to do and can be done anywhere.

I decided that I was in it for the long haul, so I was not in a hurry to get to a high number of miles per run. The priority was to start running without a lot of pain, and build miles slowly until my Bod became ready for more.

The first day, I ran one block and walked one block until I had 20 minutes in. I did this one block stuff for about two weeks, two days in a row followed by one day of rest. After two weeks I felt stronger and added

95

30 minutes, now 5 blocks at a time. I was at about the 8-week mark when I was jogging about 3 miles in 30 minutes. Within a year I was running 6 miles in 48 minutes. It was a slow buildup, but I had no injuries and running became a permanent lifestyle.

30 years later I still run, but now cross-train with biking and swimming. I exercise about 5 times a week for one hour. I space two days of rest in. The point is, there was no hurry because I did not want instant running success but rather a lasting lifestyle change. I got it and love exercising.

Row Row Row Your Fat

How many of you have a rowing machine in your basement, garage, or storage room? Exercise bike? Treadmill? Have you sold a piece of exercise equipment at a garage sale for 50 cents that is now in somebody else's basement? Figure out a way to use it that you will enjoy, such as in front of your TV. Use it or lose it.

Exercise Rule: You can out-eat your exercise, so don't exercise and then SuperSize your treats for defeat.

Fabits Can Out-Eat Exercise Any Day, Every Day

The rule is to not out-eat your exercise. Exercise may help you gain energy and lose the tired feeling. You don't need to join an expensive gym or buy fancy equipment, unless you choose to. Start walking, bending, stretching, swimming, hiking, and biking whenever possible and encourage others to join you. Sign up for a 5K. Turn on the fitness channel and try a few workouts. The more time you spend exercising, the less time you will spend eating or thinking about eating.

The trickiest thing is portion size per serving = X calories = X miles or X hours of exercise. But who eats 10 potato chips or a quarter of a cookie? A fun way to measure a serving is by the number of miles of jogging it takes to burn it off. **Yes, a can of pop or beer should tell you about 1.5 miles per beer or drink, potato chips 3 miles, doughnut or pastry 4-6 miles, etc.**

One mile of jogging burns off approximately 100 calories, depending on the jogger. **A piece of cake is no piece of cake when it becomes 5 miles of jogging.** What about cupcakes, pancakes and shortcakes? Any time you hear the word "cake," start running 5 miles immediately. Alfredo Sauce was not the name of a drunken sailor. Anything named Alfredo means jogging to avoid artery clogging. Fat Domes of whipped foams: run 7 miles. The extra-large size means run forever.

Now think about it: Would you run 4 miles to burn off a doughnut? If so, then eat it and run 4 miles to break even. Note that it takes jogging 5 miles to burn off love handles from an order of fries, and 1 mile per beer.

You have to run many miles to out-eat a pig-out pizza. It is true you can have a couple of slices, but can you stop at 2, 3, or eating the entire thing? Eat the entire pizza for a free spare tire or run a marathon to burn it off.

Once you start regularly exercising, you will change your mind and behind.

CHAPTER 24

EMOTIONS AND FEELINGS:
FAT UNAPPEALING

Fat Is Not First a Health Issue, but Rather an Emotional Issue

Moods and emotions cause thoughts, both positive and negative. Your thoughts affect your beliefs, attitudes, selection of food, and exercise. Moods and emotions dominate our thinking. When we are in a bad mood and our thoughts become negative, we are ready to give up.

The great news is that moods and emotions can trigger and set off your Weapons of MassAssDestruction. Emotions can help make you stronger and help you fight on to fat war victory. Positive emotions trigger thoughts that power self-motivators that will help you win your desired fun-filled lifestyle. Dream it, live it.

Use Emotions As Motivators to Winning Your War on Fat

You can fear, be embarrassed, experience defeats, and still have pride. You can have the will to fight, but also a sense of humor. I encourage you to talk about your fatness in good humor as long as you display fighting pride in your War Face. You must be ashamed to be fat and want to kill the Fat Ugly that hides your Beautiful Bod. You must not be ashamed of YOU as long as you are fighting to regain your Beautiful Bod and health.

> **Don't have fear of failure, but do have fear of not trying or giving up.**

Fear of Failure

Sometimes we waste energy fearing failure. People who make the most of their lives probably have failed the most. They have gotten hurt and stumbled, but got up to fight again. They take risks and fight for their dreams. They are not afraid of failure, they are afraid of not trying. They are not as afraid of dying as they are of not living.

Other people don't take chances. They don't make the sales calls that could make them money, and tell themselves that they can't sell. These people are afraid of failure, so they give up before they try.

Recognizing your doubts and fear of failure is the first step in slaying these demons. **Fear is your friend and it can motivate. Fear can paralyze you into no action, or it can cause positive action. It can save your life.**

Fear of failure chops down willpower, positive visions, discipline, focus on success, and fuels excuses, whining and can't-do's. Fear may penalize positive actions, and so fear fear and stop it! Yes, just stop fearing, it is as simple as that. As Shakespeare once said, "To fear or not to fear, that is your choice." Okay, not a perfect quote, but you get the idea!

Fear of Fat Ugly

Everybody should fear Fat Ugly. It's not just the mirror and clothes, Fat Ugly makes you feel miserable most of the time. The fear of fat can be a weapon supplying you with motivation muscles. It can be the Gatorade for your BB decisions.

Fear of Fat Ugly can be the best motivator to win that there is. Fear it putting your Bod in a prison of ugly fat. Fear it killing you with your pick of horrific health issues like diabetes or stroke. Fat is not only ugly, it is a killer of you, your fat friends, your fat children and your fat pets.

Fear: love it, embrace it, let it motivate you. Having fear of being Fat Ugly may stop you from eating the ice cream. Fear may save your arteries and your life. Now, can you still order the SuperSizeMyButt with fries for your thighs?

Fat Ugly embarrassment is your friend for self-motivation to Win Thin.

Embarrassment Pain

Is the Fat Ugly embarrassment pain unbearable? If it is, great. If not, keep heaping on the pain as it will help set you fat free. Is eating the goodies so great as to endure the embarrassment? Think about all your pain and balance that with the feelings of Looking Good, Feeling Good 24-7. LGFG with the wonderful seasoning of high self-esteem. Having people compliment you instead of gawking at your life form of a Fat Ugly. Is the malt, the SuperSizeMyButt, the pig-out eating, and night-owl snacking worth the pain of wearing them forever? Do you want to be known as King Kong or Queen Kong, or are you ready to win your war?

The Fat Warrior's Most Embarrassing Moment

I was one of five high school sophomores to qualify for the league meet. Track meets had qualified me for this honor and I was considered the second best miler in the league. It was anticipated that the best miler who was a senior from a rival school would win. People from our town were pulling for me to be the big sophomore upset and win for our school and town.

The stands were packed with townspeople, school supporters, my parents, and girlfriend. Our track coach had laid out the strategy that gave me the best chance for upset. Because I had a strong finish and my opponent did not, I was to run a steady pace that would have me in about third place by the last lap, but with a strong final kick I could edge him out and win.

The gun went off and my heart pounded. I was right on his heels from the go, the stands cheering me, the underdog, on. I stayed right on him, abandoning the coach's plan of a steady pace with a strong finish. Instead, I was running his race at his pace. It was working perfectly until the last 200 yards when I just ran out of will and energy. I not only did not keep up with him, but guys who had never beat me passed me. My coach would not even speak to me afterwards, and I felt a total embarrassment to all my supporters. I found a ride home because I could not bring myself to get on the team bus.

I learned my lesson to focus on my run and not the race, nor my competitor. Sometimes a strong and steady pace is your best chance for victory. Many people jump the gun on diets, only to find themselves running out of will to continue an unsustainable pace. **The Fat Warriors program is not a race to place. It is a journey to a happier lifestyle that evolves from changing bad decisions into good decisions.**

> ## *Pain is temporary. Quitting lasts forever.*
> **-Lance Armstrong (1971 -). U.S. cyclist, 7-time winner of the Tour de France, and cancer survivor.**

Feel the Pain

There is a song with the theme that "women all get prettier at closing time." This is akin to drinking women pretty. I saw Toby Keith sing a song called "Runnin' Block." In the song he "take[s] one for the team," a reference to acting as wingman for a friend by being friendly to a fat woman so his friend could be alone with her pretty friend.

After the song, he toasted all the women in the audience that were thinking he was a son of a bitch. This is a good story for emphasizing that the dating pool for fat people is reduced because their weight is not. Fat people are just not the date of choice for most BBs. It shows how bad it is for fat people and the pain of looks and health problems they must endure.

You may be wearing and bearing the pain now. **The more pain you have, feeling embarrassed, ugly and hurt, the more you can turn it into self-motivation to win.** Don't forget the physical pains of being Fat Ugly--lower back, joint, knee, and hip pain. Hippo Hips eventually hurt. Can you bend over and tie your shoes without physical or emotional pain?

Feel the pain, and make the decision to change to a new lifestyle for a happier life free of pain.

> *The biggest failure is the failure to participate. Participate, play games, score, and win a new life!*

CHAPTER 25

POSITIVE SELF-TALK FOR PERMANENT WEIGHT LOSS: YOUR NEGATIVE BELIEFS PUT FAT IN YOUR BRIEFS

Before you win big you must lose big. If you are currently Fat Ugly you have the losing big down, but that losing is the inspiration needed for permanent LGFG victory.
If you think you are whipped by the whipped creams of your life, then you are. Dream of winning your personal Right Size, and you will.

Self-Talk: Atomic Fat Blaster

Your command center may be programmed to enjoy the pleasure of bigging out on Fuglies and oversized portions if you are currently FU. If you are programmed to attract Fat Ugly, your Self-Talk can deprogram and reprogram to attract Looking Good. **Your Self-Talk and imagery are always there for you to call on and utilize to your advantage. Self-Talk is free: no expensive plan, no contract, and no minute limit. Only one salesperson to deal with, and that is YOU!**

Your Self-Talk may tell you the pain is not great enough to give up those Fugly goodies. If so, you will eat them. Self-Talk may tell you that you can't win your war on fat. In that case, you are a doomed excuse

104

victim of Self-Talk and will not achieve Fat Warrior status. Turn in your War Face and sit on the couch, grow wide hide, and watch until you are ready to fight for your personal Right Size.

Your Self-Talk may say that conquering your Fabits is worth the benefit of getting more attention from the opposite sex. **Self-Talk may convince you to make the BB decisions that will lead you to the front lines, from spectator to participator in a fun-loving lifestyle.**

Self-Talk is a Fat Warrior weapon that Fuglies fear. No spies in the world can tap into, control or hear your Self-Talk. It is your unique and powerful weapon. People make fun of people talking to themselves, but Fat Warriors applaud Self-Talk. You Self-Talk the pounds right off your fat behind if Self-Talk directs your decisions to looking and feeling your best. **As long as you keep talking to yourself and saying you can win, you are never defeated.** Self-Talk can be the best talk you have all day!

Law of Override Depression: **Your Bod is the barometer of how you feel. If you look and feel Fat Ugly, that feeling will override to dominate your thoughts about yourself.**

When you start Looking Good and Feeling Good, that feeling will dominate your thoughts and beliefs. Your thoughts become your beliefs whether or not they are factual. What you believe you will achieve.

Your Beliefs Are True, Even If They Are Not Factual

Whatever you believe is reality for you. If you believe it or perceive it to be true, then it is a fact to you even if it is not actually true in reality.

Example: Three people see a fudge brownie with ice cream and coconut on top. One person believes he must have it, that it will provide great pleasure and that is true for him. He knows the consequences, but believes he must have it. His belief is true for him, he cannot resist, and so he eats and wears.

Second person sees the brownie and she says, "It looks good. I would enjoy a bite, and I can control my desire for it." Her belief is true for her and so she takes a bite and leaves the rest.

Third person says, "I can't believe I used to eat that junk. It made me fat and bloated. If I ate that today it would make me sick." So he leaves it on the table without touching it.

Did the brownie cause the beliefs? No, the brownie was the same in all cases, while each person thought about it differently and acted according to his or her beliefs. The brownie was simply there for all to react to.

Think about eating junk and you will eat junk, look like junk, feel like junk, with junk in your trunk.

Think about eating fresh and nutritious often and you will learn to love it and feel great.

Your Power of Think & Your Beliefs

Identify demon beliefs and the desired beliefs that you want on your team. Example of wrong belief: All the Christmas gifts make you happy. They do, but only for days or minutes. My grandson gets many new toys on Christmas, but after a week he is playing with the boxes they came in. The point is that his first belief is that the toys will make him happy, but reality sets in when it is seen how temporary they are.

The ice cream cone is temporary enjoyment, but then you have to house it forever. You have the power of think! Think the ice cream back into the cone as you leave it alone.

Change the Core Beliefs at Your Core

Scrutinize the beliefs at your core and get them in concert to help you fight to become your personal Right Size. Shed any counter-productive Self-Talk that will stop you from controlling your weight. Your positive Self-Talk and thoughts will do the rest to have you eat healthier, lose weight, keep it off, and look and feel your best.

The fact is, you can decide on the apple over the brownie via Self-Talk and beliefs. If you can choose the apple once, then you can choose it again and again. This will change your core belief and you will soon love the apple more than the brownie.

Believe to Achieve Mind Over Fatter

Lay your doubts aside and believe to achieve an LGFG lifestyle. It must be what you want most and you must visualize it. It must dominate your thoughts to empower BBs over Fuglies. Right Size with the power of Mind Over Fatter.

You will never give up because you have Pit-Bull mentality and are destined to win your war. You must have an absolute belief that you can win and will win.

That becomes your only acceptable choice. Put your War Face on, war on, read on! Mind Over Fatter. **You can do it!**

CHAPTER 26

ACCOUNTABLE ACCOUNTABILITY PARTNERS TRIM **YOU**

> *The opposite of having an excuse is accepting the blame for failure and recognizing the learning experience to make one better. This is also referred to as accepting the responsibility and consequences of your behavior. If you do this, then you have more power to change and win your BB.*

Accept Blame, Don't Blame

Shame beats the hell out of blame. Blame is for people who can't cut it because it is easier to blame than achieve.

You can't delegate the responsibility of your Bod to anybody. Have the accountability for it. Don't try to delegate it to diets, pills, meals on wheels, shakes, or fat blasters. Their responsibility is to their bottom line and not to your bottom.

Accountability Partners Mean Success

Enlist your spouse, friend or family member to hold you accountable and encourage you. Be careful, though, as sometimes those closest to us have been our enablers in the past. Because they love us, it can be difficult for them to call us out when we are straying from our plan. **If that's the case, seek support with**

Fat Warriors members at www.lifestyleweightexperts.com.

Having an accountability partner means rising to challenges. Accountability partners make sure responsibility is taken for FU and BB decisions, and you can push each other to meet set goals.

Also try forming an accountability team! With an accountability team, you can compete with and challenge your teammates. See who wins the title of Scoring Champions. Play scoring games and compare personal records!

CHAPTER 27

POSITIVE STEPPING TO BECOMING A LIFETIME RIGHT SIZE

Use Social Media to Tell Others!

Do you have a Facebook and/or MySpace page? Blog? Twitter? Are you linked in on LinkedIn? Social media sites are a great way to get people involved in Fat Warriors and to keep others up to date on your progress. By blogging or posting updates on your media pages, you can include your family and friends in your fight against Fat Ugly. This can be a helpful source of support and encouragement that will help you win your LGFG lifestyle!

Brag Session

Once a day, think about things you appreciate about you. Be creative and be thankful. There is so much more to be thankful for. Giving yourself five compliments every morning takes about 25 seconds and lasts all day. So smile and think about all the wonderful qualities you have. Believe in yourself and focus on making things happen!

Help Others Learn and You Will Benefit More

It is known that when we help others we help ourselves. As a Fat Warrior, by helping others fight fat you will help yourself. As a professional speaker and author, I know that I will learn more than my audience or readers because of the research, dedication and preparation needed before writing and speaking.

By teaching others, I continue to benefit in my own life through the reinforcement of the Fat Warrior principles. Try it! It works for me, and it will work for you!

Get Connected to Positive Support Groups

Have you noticed smokers hang with smokers and nonsmokers hang with nonsmokers? Often times fatties hang with other fatties, and thins hang with thins. Your support groups will help determine your success or failure in reaching your Right-Sizing goal.

You can choose groups that support Right Sizing, healthy lifestyles and making BB decisions:

- Role models: mother, father, brothers, sisters, friends.
- Meetings or clubs (lifestyleweightexperts.com).
- Focus on positive people to influence your eating and exercising.
- Get a personal trainer, coach, or friend to help you and be your check stand watcher, decisions helper and supporter!

Enthusiastic Connections from Other People and Organizations

Getting connected to the right groups will give you amazing support and encouragement. Success is tied to the support and recognition by friends, enemies, relatives, and anybody.

Order the Fat Dome in the presence of BB people or make Fugly decisions and they will tell you about it. Get connected to the right groups that will give you truth, support, help, and encouragement. Seek out enthusiastic connections from other people and organizations.

Fact: Chatter Melts Fat Away!

Chatter on a baseball diamond is when the players chatter encouraging talk to each other. It really helps support the pitcher if you are on defense. If offense, chatter to the batter gives encouragement. Mental chatter/cheering or talking positively helps people perform.

Chatter matters, so cheer your BB averaging and your improvements to friends. Team up for chatter over fatter. Talk about wins and how to improve losses. Compete, team up, and have fun winning. Twitter, Facebook, MySpace, FatBook or ...?

Have Can-do Attitude

Positive people are the people who succeed. Just look around, who has accomplished anything whining about life? Positive people are more successful, so which do you choose to be?

Positive changes may not be seen today, but they can start today. Healthy change must be a long-term process. Having a can-do attitude instead of negativity can start you on your way to your new TrimStyle lifestyle.

Fat Warrior on Your Shoulder

Summon the Fat Warrior at any time for encouragement and support. This fat war is fought by the Fat Warriors Nation and YOU. You have the Fat Warrior on your shoulder that you can take with you 24-7. Winning your fat war relies on you, and you can get support from the Fat Warriors Nation!

Picture Perfect

Carry a picture of yourself when you were BB or close to it. Look at it when you get ready to make an FU decision. Carry a split photo--one side before, one side fatter. Now, will you buy that fudge sundae?

You must weigh the good feelings of 10 minutes of eating pleasure against the pain of shame and being fat 24-7. You decide which one you want.

Naysayers Suck!

Naysayers don't do and they discourage doers. They are purveyors and perverts of the discipline and will to succeed. Naysayers suck! They suck the will out of people around them and perpetuate the comfort of failure by discouraging the possibilities of success.

Just stay away from naysayers and tell them they have negative karma that Fat Warriors do not team with. Show them your War Face and tell them you are a winner. Like baseball, you are trading them for a positive friend.

<u>Law of Look Like Your Friends</u>: You become what your friends are and eat what they eat. If your friends are oinkers, you are likely a pig.

You Mirror Your Friends

See a gang of friends who are fat and see fat hanging all over them. Fat friends love to order fat foods. They protect each other from feeling bad about French fries, ice cream, Fat Domes, etc. They allow each other to feel good feeling bad.

You mirror your friends. You look like them, dress like them, eat like them. If your friends do lots of shots you are probably a six-shooter; if they don't, you do not understand this sentence.

Hang around with fat people? If the friends you hang around with are fat, fat will hang on you. I hung around with smokers and became one. Ditto on drinking, cussing, etc. The good news was that my friends also had a lot of positive traits, and I picked up those, too.

If you want to eat healthy and look good, hang around with people that look good and eat healthy. The Lifestyle Weight Experts Team does not suggest that you ditch your friends if they are fat, only that you become more aware of your behavior when you are with them. Maybe there are more positive people you can hang with who can influence and encourage you to keep fighting for a more healthy lifestyle.

> *Everything is relationships, so ship out with people that are on your desired BB lifestyle voyage.*

CHAPTER 28

MORE FAT WARRIORS
SKINNY THINNING
STRATEGIES

Nothing in the world can take the place of persistence. Talent will not; nothing is more common than unsuccessful men with talent. Genius will not; unrewarded genius is almost a proverb. Education will not; the world is full of educated derelicts. Persistence and determination alone are omnipotent. –Calvin Coolidge

7 BBs of Highly Effective Hot Bods:
1. Eating to live, not living to eat
2. Scoring and Averaging FUs & BBs
3. Decision Accountability
4. Eating Naked: stripping processed foods from your diet
5. Right-Sized Portions
6. Practicing the 7:30 Rule and 20-Minute Rule
7. Exercising

7 Fabits of Self-Sabotaging Fat Ugly Bods:
1. Diet and Scale-aholics
2. Unaware of consequences of decisions
3. Excuses Victims
4. Night Commando Eating
5. Portion Pigs

6. Sweet treats for rewards
7. Too tired to exercise today, maybe tomorrow

Begin With Your Fat End in Mind

In the book *The Seven Habits of Highly Effective People*, author Stephen R. Covey says to begin with the end in mind. He is not talking about BUTTS, but rather that you must dream, vision and plan with the end result in mind. Your desired tight end might have you planning and dreaming of enjoying life with full participation, instead of living life with deprivation. **You must begin with your tight end in mind.**

If you think and believe that you will always be fat, then you lose and you will be.

Can You Think Yourself Thin?

You absolutely can think yourself thin or you will think yourself into Fat Ugly. It is that simple, your thinking drives your thoughts. Your thoughts become your beliefs. Your beliefs, either true or false in actuality, are always true to you.

Your thoughts will guide the Big 4 Fat Makers or 4 Thin Makers: the fork, the spoon, the glass, and the hand. Your decisions will determine your Fat Bod or Hot Bod lifestyle.

Your war on fat is won or lost before it ever begins. If you think long enough whether you will eat the banana split, it will soon be splitting your jeans size. You will eventually eat it. Think about that. You start eating Fat Ugly long before you become fat. Think about why that is true. So have Pit-Bull attitude, put on your War Face, growl, bare your teeth, and scare Fabits to win BB!

Confidence is used by winners in business, writing, speaking, and especially in sports. In sports they sometimes refer to an athlete's problems as "between his ears." That usually means the athlete is doubting and lacks confidence. As an ex-pitcher, a businessman, author, and speaker, I know that confidence is an absolute must to be a winner at anything. Confidence and beliefs are not options, they are musts. Confidence is so important that it was inducted into the Hall of BB Fame after being named a Top Ten WMAD!

Time: Your Vicodin for the Pain of Change

Giving up a bad Fabit is PAINFUL. Time is the Vicodin for the pain of change. Think of your bad Fugly Fabits keeping you from your personal Right Size.

As you stop the Fugly Fabits and keep making BB decisions, **at first you will experience pain, but time will be your Vicodin as you become pain free.** Stop eating after 7:30 p.m., and the pain will be intense for about 30 days. Then the pain diminishes and soon it will be your new painless lifestyle. That improvement will add a high of pride. **Eating after 7:30 p.m. is so fat horrendous that it made the Fat Ugly Hall of Shame.**

With time as your Vicodin, you can eliminate the pain of the Fabit and be pain free in about 30 days as your new BB lifestyle becomes the new you. Think over a year of what kicking a few Fabits will mean to you in Body, Mind, and Spirit!

Stop Speed-Eating and Oinking

Eating fast until you're stuffed, puffed out, and one belt buckle past full results in Stupid Fat. You engorge yourself with food fast, and now that you're stuffed you bloat up with an added dessert. That fat gut will expand to accommodate as you fork it in. You must have slower chew time for a better waistline.

Instead of your current FatStyle, you can change to a new TrimStyle that you will love yourself for doing. This principle will work, but you must participate for 30 days. Once again, that 30-day change of behavior thing works! Quit thinking about it and commit or sit on the porch. Win this Fabit to BB and wear your slow-eating Hot Bod into a smaller size.

Observe a Speed-Eater Oinking to Stop Forever!

Notice fork to mouth speed and cheeks blown out to hold maximum food. Head back for the big gulp down. By the time a Speed-Eater's stomach relays the message that it is full, it's too late because they ate the plate. **If you are a Speed-Eater, put the shovel down, breathe, converse, and chew your food. Simply slow down and you will come down in clothing size.**

If you're not in a hurry to get fat, eat slowly you will be able to leave the table satisfied instead of stuffed and feeling miserable. Stuffed full feels like tired and bloated; satisfied feels great with energy. Another phenomenon will occur: You will actually enjoy your meal. You will find that food is not in a hurry to leave the plate, it will wait for you. Leave the table stuffed and puffed (FU) or satisfied with the feeling of energy by eating proper portions (BB).

Don't Do the Stuff, Wallow, and Swallow

You know what looks uglier than fat? A fat full mouth doing the Stuff, Wallow, and Swallow. Like speed dating, the Stuff, Wallow, and Swallow almost skips the chewing. Watch this phenomenon in action and you will stop doing it.

119

Posture Defeats Fat and Depression

Studies show that posture affects your confidence, your fight, even your attitude.

Drill sergeants make recruits stand at attention and march with shoulders back and chin up. Why did your parents always tell you to straighten up and don't slouch? When people see someone slumped over with round shoulders and chin down, they often see a gloomy person. The same people who see a person with shoulders back and chin up see confidence. Posturing is constantly used by winners. How about the gorilla and chest thumping--that is a form of posturing. The fact is, when your back is straight and your chin is up, you are more likely to win your personal Right Size and even career challenges.

There are neurons and substances released in the Bod that show that people perform better and feel better when they have good posture. Accept that posture can help drive Fugly decisions down. The right posture can posture you into more BB decisions. This simply means posture can help build your dream lifestyle with confidence.

Use every tool at your command to feel great and win. Throw your shoulders back and march to your victories. Gain swagger instead of fat!

Mix it Up!

One common reason for relapse is that your routine has become too, well, *routine*. Find a new, healthy recipe to try. Then go shopping at a different store or farmers' market, bring home some new healthy ingredients, and have some fun in the kitchen. Take a new exercise class or a new walking route. Make it new and interesting again. **Watch for interesting recipes on our website at www.lifestyleweightexperts.com.**

Be Your Bod's CEO

Your Bod is your Company and you are the President and CEO. You run your Bod, it does not run you. Your decisions decide what you want your Bod to look and feel like. Your Bod will always perform like YOU run it, powered by your decisions and lifestyle. **Your Bod never makes a mistake and reacts perfectly to your commands.**

Staying fat is your decision. Gaining your personal Right Size is your decision. It is your decision and lifestyle, and YOU rule!

Hire Your Food

Like a job, food can be given a job description and interview. You can also give the foods you eat a performance appraisal to see if they are doing their job. **If the foods you eat are causing Fat Ugly depression, loss of job, loss of dates, creating avoidance, and self-loathing, fire them!** They may taste good, but may also be causing you poor health and misery. If the foods you eat are fresh, organic, nutritious foods that are performing well by giving you confidence, promote them, give them a raise, and eat more of them!

Food can also be hired on a part-time basis. I personally love French fries, and I do mean *love*. I especially like them hidden in a cheeseburger basket with ketchup all over them. I do not hire the cheeseburger basket as a full-time food, instead I hire the fatbasket now and then.

Performance Management

You can track the performance of the foods you eat by ScoreBooking daily, doing weekly comparisons, and by comparing monthly and annual progress. Food must have a successful track record of keeping your Bod Looking Good, Feeling Good, and the proof is on your ScoreCard.

CHAPTER 29

EATING CULTURE + FRIENDS
=
FAT OR THIN

Emotional and Social Land Mines

Food isn't just used to satisfy hunger, it is also a common part of social interactions and a means of comfort and stress relief. How we eat is also partially dictated by how we were raised. "Clean your plate!" or "There are starving people in Africa!" are some of the phrases we've all heard growing up. What's a healthy eater to do?

First, consider how and when you eat. Do you only eat when you're hungry, or do you reach for snacks while watching TV or hanging out with friends? Do you eat when you are stressed or bored? Do you use food to reward yourself? **Recognizing your personal culture and emotional triggers can make it easier for you to make positive changes. Once you realize your own personal challenges, you can work towards gradually changing the mental attitudes that have sabotaged your efforts.**

Biggest Influences on Your Eating

What are the biggest influences on your eating-- McDonald's, the government, Mommy, Daddy, emotions, Fugly foods, movie stars, athletes, school, or teachers? As a Fat Warrior, you don't need a nutritionist or diet expert to tell you the following: Eating ice cream, candy bars, doughnuts, cake, pies, salad dressings, and French fries will make you fat, dam your arteries, and bake your self-esteem.

Culture Questions

- Why do so many people love their lifestyles of exercise, while others hate the thought of breathing heavy?
- Why can some people quit smoking and others can't?
- Why do some people eat to be Fat Ugly and others prefer healthy eating?
- Why can some people quit drugs and others can't?
- Why can some people quit alcohol and others can't?

They all have a commonality, they are killing themselves or making themselves better. Some people change and others do not, according to the culture of their lives. I wonder how many are just afraid to start, and so they never see the journey with rewards and fun. **People are afraid to start because their culture demons keep them from the start line.** Look for your angels and you will be ready to run your race.

Fat Ugly Thought Provokers Provided by Our U.S. Culture:

- School menus loaded with fat food choices and pop
- TV ads with images of skinny people eating fat foods
- Fataurants with fast food where you can eat and drive while talking on your cell phone and sending a text message
- All-you-can-eat stuffets, also instantly ready foods. Just pile, pay and chomp for $9.95
- Images of hot fudge sundaes with nuts and whipped cream and other fat treats. Where is the carrot? Oh yes, it's in the carrot cake with vanilla frosting.

> *Our river of thoughts is polluted by these images unless we control the river. The good news is YOU CAN.*

Your Bod Today

Your Hot Bod does not exist today because of fate or what you ate. Your Bod today exists because of a river of Fabit thoughts always flowing through your mind. **Your river of thoughts floods your brain with a strong current of Fugly decision power that puts your Bod into FU action.** You can't dam the river, but you can control the currents of thoughts that put your Bod decisions into action. Control the thought river and you will control your Bod size. The lifeguards of discipline, desire, and willpower all swim in the river and are ready to help you.

The most important thing is to think about yourself and what your life will be like encased in Fat Ugly forever and ever and ever. That many evers is a long time, and in a very short while you can start changing your behavior and create your dream scenario that you believe will come true. It can come true if you believe. Live the dream to make it happen.

Control the River - Change Your Appetite

Changing your appetite is like changing any habit. It takes time, but only weeks. After a while, I noticed that I craved my favorite Fuglies less and less until they were almost wiped from existence and from my Bod. I now like healthier foods and the Fuglies have lost most of their appeal. I will occasionally consume Fuglies, but Captain Crave is no longer ordering me to eat them. I am at peace with a piece of cake. Control your thought river to control your waistline.

Who's Driving Your Appetite Bus?

Riddle: Which came first, the appetite bus driving the eating decisions or the eating decisions driving the appetite bus? **Answer:** Does it matter? You must understand that your decisions drive your appetite bus. Your appetite bus is driven by your culture. You could successfully argue that the physiology of being hungry drives the appetite bus and you would win a merit badge.

The Fat Warrior is only speaking of choices, not hunger pains. When you are hungry, eat, but let decisions drive your hunger to an appetite for *healthy* foods.

CHAPTER 30

FAT WARRIORS DON'T QUIT
AND
GET FUN FIT

> *The credit belongs to the man who is actually in the arena; whose face is marred by dust and sweat and blood; who strives valiantly; who errs and comes short again and again; who knows the great enthusiasms, the great devotions, and spends himself on a worthy cause.* –Theodore Roosevelt

When the FU Bull Bucks You Off, Get Back Up on the Decisions Saddle

Cowboys know that they will be bucked off the bull many times, but the champions all get back in the saddle to ride again. Getting bucked off or knocked down in favor of FUs will not lead to defeat, but **not getting up and fighting again <u>will</u> lead to certain defeat.**

The baseball player knows he will get hit by many pitches and knows the pain. The player knows that only if he gets back in the box will he be in a position to hit the home run.

Relapse

Alcohol and drug rehab programs know that it usually takes the completion of more than one program, and many people relapse. The fact is that if people don't give up, they eventually realize the emotional and physical pain of their addictions proved to be the impetus to finally win their addiction battle.

The winning battle strategy is to not embrace these minor setbacks and delays, but see them as part of the process. You get tackled many times before you get into the end zone.

You will start by making some decisions. Keep good decisions up and you will experience a change of habit. The change of habit will evolve into a lifestyle change, and that is when you have won. Just keep your momentum going, don't give up if you stumble, and you will win your race.

I have learned that in business, sports, and life that you are still winning as long as you are trying and fighting. You are the loser only when you give up and let Fat Ugly win.

Relapse is not collapse. Score BBs, average and win your personal Right Size.

> *Remember, you don't win a war without losing*
> *some battles first.*

Recommit, Don't Quit

You may become discouraged and think you can't do it. Never quit, instead *recommit*. Resume ScoreBooking. **You cannot lose if you are determined to fight and score.** It may take many attempts and time, but it is a necessary process for improving what is necessary for victory. Experiencing some failures is normal, but you will get back up and keep striving so you will win in the long run.

Don't take the road disguised as easy. I can't think of one thing that is easy about being Fat Ugly. Dating, jobs, breathing, moving, tying your shoe laces. Can you bend down and tie your shoe laces?

CHAPTER 31

YOUR FAT WARRIORS CHALLENGE

Fast Food Challenge

McDonald's saw the Fat Warriors coming, so their math indicates. They added salads and subtracted trans fats. They have, and are, creating many healthy choices. Kudos to Mickey D's, the Fat Warriors salute your progress. You decide what gets loaded onto your spoon and fork, so fork up to your best interests at McD's.

McDonald's and other fast food places have some excellent choices, just don't big out on the bad ones. Make BB menu choices. Show yourself, your friends, and family that you can make Beautiful Bod decisions at many Fataurants. Make a game of it with your kids, **the Can-Do Challenge**. Your family can eat grilled chicken salads and watch the oinkers SuperSize themselves. These observations will have a dynamic impact on you and your kids. Observing what waddlers order will give you and your children insight to find the problem and answer in one word. It is not calories, foods, SuperSizeMyButt portions, or trans fats, but rather **decisions**. You can make BBs or Fuglies. It's your choice.

Take someone to lunch at a fast food Fataurant and order a healthy choice. Eat it while watching how the fatties eat and say, "That used to be me." You will feel great as you watch Hippo Hips order the SuperSizeMyButt fat baskets with cheeseburgers and fries while you are eating healthy.

Warriors stay away from SuperSizing their hips with their lips. Say NO to SuperSizeMyButt meals and YES to baked, broiled, or grilled lean meat, fish, salads, soup, and whole grains.

Fat Warriors Against Fat

We are at war against Fat Ugly and its effect on people. You are now beginning your war, and it will become your new, positive way of life. When you are LGFG, everything is more fun and life is beautiful. You are more attractive to the opposite sex, you are better in business, may make more money, and feel better around your children and significant other. You will be wearing happy smiles instead of Fugly frowns.

With the Fat Warriors program, there are no guarantees because we do not sell miracle pills or magic elixirs. **However, we do guarantee, and your judgment tells you, that if you make the right decisions you will win your war on fat and make your Right-Size goal a reality**.

We guarantee that Fat Warriors will be in your face and will war with you as our army helps you defeat Fat Ugly. We guarantee that you can put on your special War Face, give your Combat Growl, and start making BBs now!

It costs your Bod and your pocketbook to be Fat Ugly. Be hard on your fat and order it off your Bod. Demand that fat leave you alone forever. Will it to leave, and then make the decisions to make it happen.

Life Is Too Short to Live It Fat Ugly

As you record on your ScoreCard, keep in mind that mastering this lifestyle change is an ongoing adventure. On the scales of life, you will lose fat pounds as you gain fat-fighting momentum and self-esteem. We congratulate you on taking this journey to become your personal Right Size. You now may join the Fat Warriors Nation.

Our mission throughout the Fat Warriors program is to make this challenging journey of

changing behavior as fun as possible. We hope that this is one of the reasons that you are continuing the fight for your permanent Best Bod.

There is nothing that can prevent you from succeeding in gaining your Right-Sized Beautiful Bod for life. Fat mines and FU traps are all over, but now you are equipped with tools to help disarm those ugly fat invaders and diverters. You understand that you can pre-plan your attack method and be victorious. Make sure you reward yourself for the victories you have accomplished.

Become a Fat Warriors Recruiter--recruit your friends, family, kids and grandchildren, and have fun fighting fat and making people happy!

Please Visit Our Website at www.lifestyleweightexperts. com

Fat Warriors Nation Needs Your Stories!

We need our readers to send us stories for future Lifestyle Weight Experts books. Examples: **Fat Warriors Top Fat Ugly Stories** (what I did wrong, fat horror stories, this could happen to you stories, bad things that happen when you are fat stories, your Top Ten Fabits, your top BB suggestions, etc.). We want **100 ideas for lifestyle changes that make a positive difference.** We also need **100 fat failures,** as those stories are also highly impactful. **Send us your stories today, and they may end up in our books and seminars!**

Please share your **success stories and fat defeats** so that others may learn from your experiences. We appreciate your **experiences and advice to which parents and children can relate. Photos are welcome** only with your written permission to make public. We will not return photos or materials.

Your tips will help other people win their wars on Fat Ugly. Your stories and ideas will educate and inspire others, and may even save lives.

We also want **ideas for contests, challenges, tests, and attack fat war games, like Fattleship.** What games would you suggest? Be creative!

Your stories must be things that you want to share with the public and become the property of Lifestyle Weight Experts. Send to **www.lifestyleweightexperts.com.** If you wish to remain anonymous, do not sign your name. On the other hand, if you wish to sign your name and give permission to take your information into public venues, please supply your contact information. In both cases, we need your written permission to publish.

The Lifestyle Weight Experts Team welcomes you to the Fat Warriors Program. You will put on your War Face, and someday put the sunroof down and drive out in your new best Hot Bod!

Watch for Other Lifestyle Weight Experts Books and Products at www.lifestyleweightexperts.com

Books & eBooks

Don't Blame McDonald's, Did Mommy Make You Fat? First in the Fat Warriors series. Find out why calorie counting and diets don't work, and how ScoreAveraging changes your thoughts to change your jeans size.

Die Dieting or Lose Weight for Life: How you can develop mind control to pilot your thoughts into your Best Bod and lifestyle.

Eating Naked: The Fat Warriors guide to scrumptious eating based on recipes and meals stripped of their chemicals and additives. Projected release date TBA.

Parents--Role Models or Dough Models: Helps parents with the role of raising Right Sized, healthy children, and avoiding setting examples that will result in fat children and pain. Anticipated release date TBA.

Interact with the Fat Warriors Nation

Lifestyle Weight Experts Boot Camps, Seminars, and Speeches: See our website at www.lifestyleweightexperts.com.

FAT WARRIORS GLOSSARY

BB: Short for **Body Beautiful, Beautiful Bod, Best Bod**.

BB Average: Your Beautiful Bod or Best Bod Average. To calculate your BB Average, take your total number of BB decisions and divide by your total number of BB and FU decisions.

BB Decisions: Decisions to eat **Beautiful Bod** foods that will help you attain your Best Bod permanently, like eating an apple instead of a piece of cake. A decision to exercise is a BB.

Big Out: Over-indulging in food.

Beautiful Bod ("BB"): Your **Beautiful Bod** is a result of your **Beautiful Bod** decisions.

BMS: Refers to the trinity of Bod, Mind, and Spirit. All three must be in concert to reach your goal of attaining your personal Right Size.

Cheat-Eating: Like cheating on your significant other, if you do it, you know it when you chew.

Cognitive Dissonance: The difference between the Bod you have and the Bod you want.

Combat Growl: You will earn and learn yours.

Date Plate: Splitting a restaurant meal between two people, even dessert.

DietHolic: Person who is continually on a diet. DietHolics lose weight, only to suffer rebound pounds and start a new diet.

Eating Naked: Strip chemicals, eat organic.

Fabit: A Fat Ugly habit, such as night snacking.

FantaSize: Positive visions of how and what you want your Bod and lifestyle to be, such as a firmer Bod, sexy flat stomach, and LGFG lifestyle.

Fat Bullies: Ice cream, sugar cereals, no exercise, pop, etc.

FatCrap: Undesired chemicals and additives placed into foods.

Fat Dome: Coffee house drinks with domes of whipped cream, chocolate, and other sugar-laden toppings.

Fat Five: Like being included as someone's "Fab Five" phone contacts, Fat Five refers to your goal of planning for five FU decisions per month.

FatStyle/FatStyling: Your current lifestyle of Fat Ugly.

Fat Tax: Tax that politicians would place on fat.

Fat Ugly ("FU"): The Ugly look of obesity. You know it when you see it and when you wear it.

Fat Warrior: What you will become by making decisions to attain your Best Bod. You will work your way up through the ranks. Join us, team up, and defeat fat!

Fataholic: Person who believes he or she is condemned to Fat Ugly because of an addiction to the taste pleasures of Fugly foods.

Fataurants: Fast food restaurants serving up tasty Fugly foods.

FatCorn: Popcorn laden with huge amounts of creamy butter.

FatCrap: Undesired additives and chemicals placed into processed foods. FatCrap is an ugly name for ugly chemicals.

Fatting Average: Your Fat Ugly or FU Average. To calculate your Fatting Average, take your total number of FU decisions and divide by your total number of BB and FU decisions.

FU: Short for **Fat U**gly.

FU Decision: A **F**at **U**gly decision that makes one fat, such as eating a brownie or TV-couching and crunching.

Fugly/Fuglies: Slang relating to Fat **U**gly or **FU**.

Grabits: Grocery carts filled with Fabits are called Grabits.

Hogger: Another term for a Fat Ugly person. A waddler.

Hot Bod (Body): Your best possible Bod that you will pay the price for and earn. This does not mean movie-star hot, but your realistic personal best Bod for looks and health.

Joke Coke: Sugar-laden soda that often accompanies a SuperSizeMyButt meal as if it is free, but comes with about 300 calories.

Law of Attraction: Theory that what you envision, think about, talk about, and associate with becomes reality in time. If you constantly think about Fat Ugly foods and weight gain, that will become your reality.

Law of Fattraction: Fat Warriors theory that if you think about fat, you will attract Fat Ugly.

LG: Short for Looking Good.

Looking Good, Feeling Good ("LGFG"): Lifestyle of self-esteem and joy when you are winning your war from FU to LG.

Mind Over Fatter: Using your mind to help you choose not to eat a Fugly.

MochaChocaLatte: Coffee drink loaded with tasty fat pleasures.

Mousing: Raiding the fridge in the middle of the night.

Pit-Bull Mentality: Total can-do attitude and determination to defeat fat. You will never give up because you have Pit-Bull mentality and are destined to win your war against Fat Ugly.

Pork Up: Gaining Fat Ugly.

Pyramids of Lifestyle Change: Begin pyramiding at the bottom and baby step up the Fat Warriors Pyramids of Lifestyle Change to the level you feel comfortable with.

Rebound Fat (a/k/a Rebound Pounds): Gaining Fat Ugly back, along with horrible depression plus the avoidance factor, after dieting.

Right Size/Right Sizing: Achieving the personal size and weight that is best for you.

Scale Tossing: Tossing scales in the trash or to a neighbor (at least into the closet for you to bring out once per month). Scale tossing can be fun when you toss a perfectly good scale to your neighbor. Then explain the Fat Warriors strategy behind scale tossing.

ScoreBook/ScoreBooking: Keeping an ongoing record of BB and FU decisions. From this record you can calculate your BB Average and Fatting Average. ScoreBooking is the best way to tell if you are improving, winning or losing.

ScoreCard: An individual page or entry in your ScoreBook.

ScoreAveraging: Using your ongoing record of BB and FU decisions to calculate your BB and Fatting Averages.

Self-Talk: What you say to yourself, composed by your thoughts, that may become your beliefs.

Speed-Eater: Speed-Eaters do the Stuff, Wallow, and Swallow, and practically skip chewing their food.

Stand-Snacking: Snacking or eating standing up.

Stuffet: Another word for an all-you-can-eat buffet restaurant.

SuperSizeMyButt: Ordering the economy-sized version of a Fat Ugly, calorie-laden meal of FU food, such as a huge cheeseburger, extra-large fries, and Joke Coke.

TrimStyle/TrimStyling: The dream lifestyle you can have when you win your war on Fat Ugly.

TV-ing: The art of eating and watching TV without awareness.

Waddler: Another term for a Fat Ugly person. A hogger.

War Face: Your personal determination mode to win your war against fat. The face you make to show that you are determined to stand your ground and fight Fat Ugly.

Weapons of MassAssDestruction (WMAD): Your brain, decisions, self-motivation, discipline, emotions, beliefs, accountability, and lifestyle changes form your arsenal against Fat Ugly.

YogaLight: Quick mental concentration for winning Right-Sizing decisions by visualizing.

FAT WARRIORS
RULES & LAWS

Electric Menu Board Rule: If you order a meal from an electric menu board and receive it in less than five minutes, you are ordering fast fat food that should come with an exercise mat and personal trainer.

Exercise Rule: You can out-eat your exercise, so don't exercise and then SuperSize your treats for defeat.

Fat Warriors Law: The chances of winning your personal war on fat are directly proportional to your pain levels of owning Fat Ugly. The higher your pains of being fat, the higher your chances of defeating FU permanently. Understanding the embarrassment you feel, the scariness of facing health issues, and the thought of not being a good dating or mating prospect will help you fight back. The more these things hurt, the more they motivate you to fight and defeat. So put on your War Face, growl, and fight your Fuglies!

Fat Warriors Awareness Rule: If you are not aware of your FU decisions, then you will wear them and have to SuperSize your clothes.

Fat Warriors Rule: Reduce your Fuglies to reduce your waistline.

Large Portion Rule: Eating large portions at any time makes the stomach full, but your brain may not get the message until 20 minutes later. This gives you time to stuff the stomach uncomfortably full. Loosen that belt; unbutton those jeans. If it curves out, then you will fill out. If you eat thin, the stomach stays in.

Law of Attraction: The Law of Attraction is a theory that what you envision, think about, talk about, and associate with becomes reality in time. It is like the movie "The Secret." What you visualize you will attract. Visualize healthy and you will attract healthy. Visualize driving your Best Bod and it will lead you to the Winner's Circle. Think about and visualize Looking Good, Feeling Good, and it will happen. Law of Attraction will help you battle fat.

Law of Dating Pool: Your dating pool is reduced in direct proportion to the amount of fat you've produced.

Law of Fattraction: Just as the Law of Attraction says that what you think about will come to you, if you are distracted from your goal by constantly thinking about the pleasures of Fugly foods you will attract Fat Ugly. This is the Fat Warriors Law of *Fattraction*. Visualize fat and you will attract fat.

Law of Forever Fat: The pleasure of temporary taste is stronger than my will to make good decisions. Therefore, I will wear the temporary fat pleasure and live with the fat lifestyle of depression, embarrassment, and bad health forever.

Law of Look Like Your Friends: You become what your friends are and eat what they eat. If your friends are oinkers, you are likely a pig.

Law of Override Depression: Your Bod is the barometer of how you feel. If you look and feel Fat Ugly, that feeling will override to dominate your thoughts about yourself. When you start Looking Good and Feeling Good (LGFG), that feeling will dominate your thoughts and beliefs. Your thoughts become your beliefs whether or not they are factual. What you believe you will achieve.

Law of Slow Is Faster: The amount of time it takes for you to take weight off quickly may be approximately the amount of time it will take you to gain it back. The slower it comes off, the longer it stays off. You are not in a hurry to Right Size. Your only focus is making decisions for permanent lifestyle changes.

Lost and Found Rule: I lost the fat, but fat found its way back in the same massive places.

One Rules: One good decision, one less sweet treat, one BB meal, one day at a time, to a better life.

Reversal of Taste Rule: Some good foods will not taste as good as fat foods at first, but the longer you eat healthy, the more you acquire a taste for healthy foods. The great news is that your taste buds will eventually lose their zest for the intense taste of fat foods.

Most good foods taste good and make you feel even better. Good foods promote health and happiness; bad foods promote high blood pressure, diabetes, low self-esteem, sad clothes, and other bad things. What is your choice for life?

Rule of Negative Decisions: When I make a negative decision, I feel bad. The more I make, the worse I feel.

Rule of Positive Decisions: When I make a positive decision, I feel good. The more I make, the better I feel.

Rule of Taste: "If it tastes good, then I must have one or treat myself to one." In a matter of minutes, the good taste is gone, and the bad feelings linger, as does the fat, forever. You wear and carry what you eat. For minutes fat foods taste real good, but make you feel bad for hours.

Small Plate Rule: Big Plate means more taste but added feelings of stuffiness. Small Plate means a comfortably full, flat stomach, and Beautiful Bod pride. The flat stomach lasts. The enjoyment of a stuffed, fat stomach is over quickly and turns to sluggish depression. It is your choice. Go happy, go LG, go Right Size.

The 7:30 Rule: Don't eat anything after 7:30 p.m. If you absolutely must, eat an apple.

The 20-Minute Rule: Don't eat until stuffed. Instead, stop when comfortable, wait 20 minutes, and see if you still want more.

Breinigsville, PA USA
11 October 2010
247094BV00004B/1/P